Dieting

Auriana Ojeda, *Book Editor*

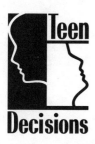

Daniel Leone, *President*
Bonnie Szumski, *Publisher*
Scott Barbour, *Managing Editor*
Helen Cothran, *Series Editor*

GREENHAVEN
PRESS®

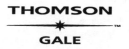

THOMSON
★
GALE

San Diego • Detroit • New York • San Francisco • Cleveland
New Haven, Conn. • Waterville, Maine • London • Munich

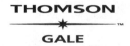

THOMSON
————*————™
GALE

For more information, contact
Greenhaven Press
27500 Drake Rd.
Farmington Hills, MI 48331-3535
Or you can visit our Internet site at http://www.gale.com

Cover credit: © David Young-Wolff/Photo Edit

LIBRARY OF CONGRESS CATALOGING-IN-PUBLICATION DATA
Dieting / Auriana Ojeda, book editor.
p. cm. — (Teen decisions)
Includes bibliographical references and index.
ISBN 0-7377-1258-9 (lib. bdg. : alk. paper) —
ISBN 0-7377-1257-0 (pbk. : alk. paper)
1. Eating disorders in adolescence. 2. Weight loss. [1. Weight loss. 2. Eating disorders.] I. Ojeda, Auriana, 1977– II. Series.
RJ506.E18 D545 2003
616.85'26'00835—dc21   2002028601

Printed in the United States of America

Contents

Foreword

The teen years are a time of transition from childhood to adulthood. By age 13, most teenagers have started the process of physical growth and sexual maturation that enables them to produce children of their own. In the United States and other industrialized nations, teens who have entered or completed puberty are still children in the eyes of the law. They remain the responsibility of their parents or guardians and are not expected to make major decisions themselves. In most of the United States, eighteen is the age of legal adulthood. However, in some states, the age of majority is nineteen, and some legal restrictions on adult activities, such as drinking alcohol, extend until age twenty-one.

This prolonged period between the onset of puberty and the achieving of legal adulthood is not just a matter of hormonal and physical change, but a learning process as well. Teens must learn to cope with influences outside the immediate family. For many teens, friends or peer groups become the basis for many of their opinions and actions. In addition, teens are influenced by TV shows, advertising, and music.

The Teen Decisions series aims at helping teens make responsible choices. Each book provides readers with thought-provoking advice and information from a variety of perspectives. Most of the articles in these anthologies were originally written for, and in many cases by, teens. Some of the essays focus on ethical and moral dilemmas, while others present pertinent legal and scientific information. Many of the articles tell personal stories about decisions teens have made and how their lives were affected.

One special feature of this series is the "Points of Contention," in which specially paired articles present directly opposing views on controversial topics. Additional features in each book include a listing of organizations to contact for more information, as well as a bibliography to aid readers interested in more information. The Teen Decisions series strives to include both trustworthy information and multiple opinions on topics important to teens, while respecting the role teens play in making their own choices.

Introduction

According to the New Zealand Health Network, 52 percent of American adolescents begin dieting before the age of fourteen. Recent studies by Anorexia Nervosa and Related Eating Disorders (ANRED) found that over half of teenage girls are dieting at any given time. The 1997 Youth Risk Behavior Study found that over 60 percent of ninth grade girls and 23 percent of ninth grade boys reported attempting to lose weight, and 80 percent of women have tried dieting before the age of eighteen. In spite of these statistics, only about 11 percent of teenagers need to lose weight according to standard height-weight charts. Thus, most teens who diet are not technically overweight or obese. You may wonder then, why do teens diet? Part of the answer is that many teens diet in reaction to the often disturbing changes that occur during puberty.

Physical Changes During Puberty

Puberty is a period of biological maturation that includes all the changes that take place when children become adults. Puberty begins when hormones—chemical substances produced by an organ, gland, or special cells that are carried in the bloodstream to regulate the activity of certain organs—prepare the body for reproduction. Puberty typically begins between the ages of eight and thirteen for girls and nine and fourteen for boys and lasts about three to four years.

The first sign of puberty in girls is breast development, which occurs at an average age of about ten-and-a-half years. Breast development is followed by a growth spurt, the growth of pubic and underarm hair, and an increase in oil and sweat production.

A girl's first period, or menarche (occurring at an average age of twelve and a half to thirteen), follows an increase in the growth of pubic hair and the external genitalia and occurs about two years after puberty begins. Around this time, a girl's body increases its stores of muscle and fat, but the ratio of muscle to fat changes from primarily muscle to equal amounts of muscle and fat. She reaches her final adult height about two years after menarche.

Puberty generally begins later in boys, at an average age of eleven and a half to twelve. Boys first notice an increase in the size of their testicles, followed later by the growth of pubic and underarm hair and an increase in penis size. They then experience a growth spurt, deepening of the voice, an increase in muscle mass, the ability to get erections and ejaculate, and the production of more oil and sweat. This is followed by the development of chest and facial hair. Boys experience their peak growth spurt about two to three years later than girls.

Puberty and Body Image

The changes that occur during puberty can affect a teenager's body image and may lead to dieting. According to marriage, family, and child counselor Judy Lightstone, "Body image involves our perception, imagination, emotions, and physical sensations of and about our bodies. It's not static—but ever changing; sensitive to changes in mood, environment, and physical experience. It is not based on fact. It is psychological in nature, and much more influenced by self-esteem than by actual physical attractiveness as judged by others. It is not inborn, but learned. This learning occurs in the family and among peers, but these only reinforce what is learned and expected culturally." Thus, body image is not just how one looks, but how one thinks, feels, and acts in response to his or her perceived appearance. Body image is closely connected with self-esteem, and it changes in response to social influences and over time.

Because girls accumulate fat during puberty, they are more likely than boys to develop poor body image and have weight concerns that lead to dieting. It is common for a young girl's self-esteem to plummet in early adolescence. Between the ages of eight and twelve, most girls gain an average of forty pounds which accumulate mainly on the breasts, hips, thighs, and buttocks. Girls who develop early are more prone to dieting and developing an eating disorder because many compare their womanly curves to their peers' childish lines and think that they are fat. These girls are more likely to try "crash" diets that involve drastically cutting calories in a short period of time and often overexercise.

Teenage boys are less likely to consider themselves overweight and in need of dieting than girls, partly because they do not typically gain a substantial amount of fat during puberty. Some boys struggle with weight loss issues, however, especially if they are teased for being overweight or if they participate in weight-restrictive sports, such as wrestling or gymnastics. Unlike many girls who diet before they are overweight, boys are likely to be moderately overweight when they begin to diet. Boys are more likely to use exercise rather than dieting as a means to lose weight, but some boys, especially athletes, adopt risky eating habits. Boys and girls often learn unhealthy eating habits from their family and peers.

Family and Peer Influence

Parents have significant influence over their teenager's body image—especially when their teens are young—and they may unintentionally encourage their teenagers to diet even if they are not overweight. Parents who have weight or body image problems themselves may pass their concerns on to their teens. If parents complain about their weight or are constantly dieting, teenagers may feel that they must watch their weight to avoid the problems that their parents are experiencing. Parents may comment on their teenagers' weight or eating habits and inadvertently wound their self-esteem and damage their body image. Some parents also become concerned over their girls' weight gain during puberty and encourage them to diet. Although the parents are trying to help, girls hear that their parents think that they are fat and may take the parents' suggestions to diet to an extreme.

Older teens are more influenced by their peers than by their parents. Teenagers place great emphasis on appearance and social acceptance, and they make significant efforts to be attractive and well-liked. If they are singled out or teased for being overweight, many teens will adopt stringent dieting practices to avoid being humiliated. Even if teenagers are not personally taunted for being heavy, they may overhear comments about other people who are overweight. In response, they may try to lose weight to ensure that they are not the object of teasing. Many teenagers feel that the best way to gain social acceptance and avoid being ridiculed by their peers is to achieve society's ideal body.

Media Influence

Teenagers learn what society considers an ideal physique primarily from the media. They are bombarded with images in magazines, movies, on television, and in music videos that decree what is fashionable and attractive. Recent studies have found that by the time a girl is seventeen years old, she has received over 250,000 commercial messages through the media. Girls see images of teen girls and women who are unrealistically thin. Experts claim that fashion models weigh 23 percent less than the average female; an average model is five feet eleven inches tall and weighs 110 pounds, while an average woman is five feet four inches tall and weighs 140 pounds. A young woman between the ages of eighteen and thirty-four has a 7 percent chance of being as thin as a catwalk model and a 1 percent chance of being as thin as a supermodel. One study found that

47 percent of the girls interviewed were influenced by magazine pictures to want to lose weight, but only 29 percent of the girls were overweight. Experts conclude that viewing images of extremely thin celebrities may negatively influence teenagers' body image and encourage them to diet.

In addition, many social critics argue that the media influences teenage boys to increase their muscle mass and build strong bodies. The current ideal male form is slender, but with broad shoulders, well-defined legs and stomach, and strong arms. Just as most girls cannot be as thin as models, most boys cannot replicate the physique they see in men's magazines, movies, and on television. The ideal male body emphasizes an absolute minimum of body fat, and teenage boys often take drastic measures to achieve this ideal. In addition to dieting and excessive exercise, some boys take anabolic steroids to increase their muscle mass. Anabolic steroids are synthetic hormones that mimic the muscle-building action of the male sex hormone testosterone. Steroids can cause impotence, shrunken testicles, breast enlargement, damage to the heart, kidneys, and liver, and halted bone growth.

The Risks of Dieting

Dieting, like steroids, can cause serious health problems for teenagers, particularly because of the acute physical changes that occur during puberty. Dieting can stunt growth because it often prevents teens from getting the calories and nutrients that they need to grow properly. If a diet does not provide enough calcium, phosphorus, and vitamin D, bones may not lay down enough calcium, which can increase the risk of osteoporosis— the progressive degeneration of bone tissue—later in life, especially in girls. Girls who diet may stop menstruating because their bodies need a certain amount of fat to maintain a regular menstrual cycle. Moreover, the absence of menstrual periods can lead to osteopenia, or low bone mass, a condition that precedes osteoporosis. Boys who diet may deprive their bodies of protein, which can prevent the proper growth of muscles.

Some experts argue that adolescent dieting can also lead to obesity. A 1999 study conducted by researchers at the University of Texas at Austin and Stanford University School of Medicine found that teenage girls who try to lose weight are more likely to gain weight, and girls who diet are three times more likely to become obese than are girls who do not diet. The researchers found that girls who diet usually start a "crash" diet that is unhealthy and extreme. When they cannot maintain such a rigid program they binge, which leads to weight gain and discouragement. Furthermore, girls who dieted excessively, took diet pills or laxatives, or binged and purged were more likely to gain weight than girls who dieted moderately.

Perhaps more seriously, extreme dieting practices are the most reliable predictors for developing an eating disorder. Eating disorders are usually indicative of family, school, or psychological problems that leave those affected feeling out of control. Choosing whether they eat gives the sufferers a sense of control over their bodies during a time when they feel they cannot control anything else. According to the Eating Disorders Association, "Eating disorders develop as outward signs of inner emotional or psychological distress or problems. They become the way that people cope with difficulties in life. Eating, or not eating, is used to help block out painful feelings. Without appropriate health and treatment, eating problems may persist throughout life." Eating disorders include anorexia nervosa (self-induced starvation), bulimia nervosa (binge eating followed by purging), and binge or compulsive eating (consuming large quantities of food in a short period of time). People with borderline eating disorders exhibit risky eating habits and an unhealthy preoccupation with food, but they are not as extreme as people with full-blown eating disorders. Anorexics and bulimics adopt dangerous practices to control their weight, such as smoking or taking drugs to control their appetites, vomiting or taking laxatives to purge their bodies, and overexercising. Over long periods of time, eating disorders can result in irregular or loss of menstruation, skin problems, irregular heartbeats, kidney and liver damage, loss of bone mass, hair loss, infertility, cardiac arrest, and death.

Obesity and Dieting Healthfully

In spite of all the risks involved, dieting can be useful if a person is truly overweight or obese. Obesity is determined by the measurement of body fat, not merely body weight. Some people might be over the weight limit for normal standards, but if they are very muscular with low body fat, they are not obese. Others might be normal or underweight, but still have excess body fat. The best single gauge for body fat is a measurement called body mass index (BMI). BMI is a ratio of a person's height to his or her weight, and it is derived by multiplying a person's weight in pounds by 703 and then dividing by the height in inches, then dividing that number by the height in inches. The result is graded on a scale to indicate levels of body fat. Federal guidelines define overweight as a BMI of 25 to 29.9 and obesity as a BMI of 30 or greater. People with BMIs above 30 are at the highest risk for diabetes, heart disease, and certain cancers. People who think that they may need to diet should see their doctor to determine if they are overweight, and if so, to help them develop a healthy diet plan.

Experts contend that more than 90 percent of people who lose weight on a diet gain the weight back within five years. Dieters usually lose weight quickly when they severely reduce their caloric intake, but they gain the weight back when they start eating normally, a phenomenon known as yo-yo dieting. Health professionals argue that this method of weight loss is not only ineffectual, but yo-yo dieting can also put people at risk for further weight gain and health complications such as heart disease and stroke. Experts maintain that the best way to lose weight and keep it off is to lose weight slowly by making long-term changes in diet and exercise.

Dieticians and nutritionists suggest that to lose weight health-fully, dieters must examine what and how much they are eating. The only way to lose weight is to decrease your caloric intake and increase your caloric output. The best way to reduce your caloric intake is to cut back on dietary sugar and fat and increase consumption of fruits and vegetables. Fruits and vegetables are low in calories, but high in healthy vitamins, minerals, and fiber, which makes you feel full. The United States Department of Agriculture's (USDA) Food Guide Pyramid, an excellent guide for a healthy diet plan, recommends that you eat three to five servings each of fruits and vegetables, two to three servings each of dairy and protein, six to eleven servings of carbohydrates, and consume fats, oils, and sweets sparingly every day.

Exercise is the best way to increase your caloric output. Experts maintain that people who exercise are more likely to keep weight off than people who do not exercise. According to professor C. Wayne Callaway, "A person not only burns calories while exercising, but if he or she is eating an adequate amount of food, calories will continue to be burned at a higher rate for up to several hours afterward." Exercise builds muscle tissue, and the more muscle tissue a person has, the more calories he or she will burn. Moreover, greater muscle mass improves the definition of a person's body and makes him or her look better and feel better. Exercise produces endorphins (feel-good hormones in the brain), boosts immunity, strengthens the cardiovascular system, reduces cholesterol, and improves self-confidence. The benefits of exercise encourage the dieter to continue exercising, which increases the likelihood that he or she will maintain a healthy weight.

The selections in this volume are aimed to enrich your understanding of the risks of dieting and the benefits of healthy weight loss. The articles in Chapter One, Reasons People Diet, discuss the pressures on teenagers to diet. Chapter Two, Eating Disorders, includes information on dangerous diseases like anorexia and bulimia. The articles in Chapter Three, How to Lose Weight Healthfully, describe healthy practices, such as exercising and choosing nutritious foods that facilitate weight loss and promote fitness. *Teen Decisions: Dieting* is meant to help you decide when dieting is necessary and provide guidance on how to lose weight safely.

Chapter 1

Reasons People Diet

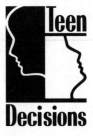

Teen
Decisions

The Media Drives Young Girls to Diet

Jessica Hendrick

In the following article, Jessica Hendrick argues that teen girls' magazines such as *Young and Modern* (*YM*) and *Cosmopolitan* cause many teen girls to diet obsessively. Teenagers who try to emulate the super-thin models in these magazines often adopt dangerous eating patterns that may turn into eating disorders. She suggests that teenagers limit their exposure to fashion magazines so that they do not view skinny models as standards to live up to. Hendrick contributes to GENaustin, a nonprofit organization that focuses on improving the self-esteem and body image of young girls.

W hen I was in junior high, I had a subscription to *Teen Magazine*. Every month I would wander through the pages of this beauty journal and pine for the look that so many of the models possessed. I would buy the products that were advertised in the magazine and follow the step-by-step instructions the magazine presented hoping to return to school the next day a changed girl.

When I was in high school I graduated to *Young and Modern*

Magazine (YM). It was the same basic routine but a more so-phisticated look. By my senior year and freshman year in col-lege, I was flipping through the pages of *Mademoiselle* and *Cosmopolitan* magazines. Overall, I would have to say that my self-image was completely hanging on whether or not I felt like I could fit into the magazine stereotype of beautiful. I'm still not there.

Thinspiration

I have friends that collect these magazines, not because of their embarrassing moments column, but for the pictures of the thin girls, because they wanted a constant reminder of how not thin they were . . . diet motivation.

In an OnHealth.com report, according to an article in the *British Medical Journal,* a study done by Australian researchers found that out of the 60 percent of teen girls who diet, one in five will develop an eating disorder. Nearly three percent of young women have a serious eating disorder. Although, no researcher has pinpointed the trigger of obsessive dieting in a majority of teen girls, the answer to me is obvious.

Media, mainly television, drives young women to near insan-ity trying to emulate the popular notion of beauty. Seeing my guy friends drool over Sarah Michelle Gellar or nearly fainting at the sight of Elizabeth Hurley makes me want to run to a plas-tic surgeon. Sometimes I don't think I can handle it. It's scary the pressure the media can put on young girls, and these teen magazines seem to offer solutions that only dig a deeper hole in self-conscience of teens.

> Out of the 60 per-cent of teen girls who diet, one in five will develop an eat-ing disorder.

I'm not saying that the media is the direct trigger of eating disorders in young women. In another OnHealth.com report, eating disorders, according to Dr. Kane, the director of the Eating Disorders program at St. Francis Medical Center in Pittsburgh, are a symptom of a personality, mental, or emotional disorder. She continues to say people with an inherited disorder will be more vulnerable to media messages, such as "thin is in." Whether or not someone develops an eating disorder, it's a well-known fact that many teenage girls struggle everyday with their self-image.

Thin Is Still In

I bought the November issue of *Teen People Magazine* the other day. I was just curious to see if anything's changed and what teen magazines are doing nowadays to ensure healthy living with all the recent statistics on teen dieting and eating disorders. Unfortunately, nothing's changed.

Taking Responsibility

"There is a fine line of responsibility on the part of the media," indicates Steven Thomsen, associate professor of communications [at Brigham Young University]. "The media do not act as an initiating, but, rather, as a perpetuating force to those who suffer from an eating disorder. To these young women who are at risk, some of these beauty and fashion magazines can be as dangerous as giving a beer to an alcoholic. The very factors that have made them vulnerable to an eating disorder also heighten their vulnerability to images of thinness and false promises of happiness."

USA Today Magazine, December 2000.

Teen People, not to rat on them but . . . is just an example of what so many teens come to for answers to self-image problems and even personal problems. "Oh, I'm not as skinny as that Jennifer Aniston. If I want to marry someone like Brad Pitt, I have to look like her. Thank God I have this teen magazine to tell me how." These magazines are more like Satan than actual help. "Ah-ha! She's come to me for answers, and I shall give her make-up tricks and diet plans that will only leave her more unhappy with herself. Ha Ha Ha!"

Okay, so that might be a bit harsh. After all, *Teen People,* like all other teen magazines, is just trying to make a buck and they've found a very effective way to do it. But, *Teen People* doesn't have to be so blunt at what they're doing. They have thirteen articles on beauty, and, out of those, half compare their beauty tips to celebrities. Page 58's article basically says, "Wanna look like Liv Tyler? Wear M.A.C. Viva Glam III lipstick." On top of that, almost exactly 50 percent of the content is advertisements for beauty products featuring thin, glamorous models. No wonder so many girls hate the way they look.

My suggestion to all you girls out there: Don't do what I did and let magazines and popular media shape the way you think you should look. Cancel your subscriptions to your teen magazines. Sure, a magazine every now and then can be helpful for health and beauty tips, but there is no reason to hate yourself every month.

Mothers Can Pressure Teenage Girls to Diet

Alison Bell

According to *Teen Magazine* contributor Alison Bell, mothers may inadvertently pressure their teen daughters to diet. Bell contends that although mothers mean well, some may comment negatively on their daughters' eating habits or be overly concerned about the natural weight gain that occurs during puberty. Most mothers do not realize how strongly they influence their daughters' self-esteem and body image, but the fact is, their comments may cause their daughters to adopt unhealthy eating practices or develop an eating disorder. In addition, mothers who diet or have had weight problems themselves may unknowingly pass their habits and negative body images on to their daughters. If you think that your mother is unnecessarily critical of your weight, Bell suggests that you talk to her about it because she may not understand how her behavior affects you.

Your mother loves you. She wants you to be confident and secure. She wants you to look and feel beautiful. Her hopes and dreams revolve around your happiness. But if your mom's all weirded out about weight issues, you may be paying the price.

Megan Sunderland remembers the first time her mom broached the subject. She was 13 and had just started her period—the "miracle of womanhood" had caused the 5-foot 6-inch Megan to blossom from 120 to 140 pounds. Already somewhat insecure about her weight— "I didn't know any other eighth graders as heavy as me, because they hadn't gone through puberty yet," she says— she would feel a lot worse, and fatter, after this particular mother-daughter chat.

> Roughly half of all teenage girls in America are on a diet.

"She told me stories about how my older sister, who's very thin, had always been able to control her eating and her weight," remembers Megan, now 16. "My mom didn't come out and say, 'Megan, you're fat.' I'm kind of sensitive, and my mom is a kind, loving person. But in my heart, I knew that's what she meant."

Not wanting to be "the fatty in the family" Megan began a drastic diet to whittle away the pounds. Eventually, she lost over 30 pounds. At her lowest point, she was a fragile 107 pounds— but she had lost more than weight; she'd lost her energy, her enthusiasm and was on the way to losing her self-esteem.

Food for Thought

Roughly half of all teenage girls in America are on a diet, according to the Seattle-based association Eating Disorders Awareness & Prevention (EDAP). Even at the age of 10, 81 percent of girls report a fear of being fat, while 51 percent report feeling better about themselves when they are on a diet.

What fuels these girls' desire to be thin? In part, however unintentional, their mothers may be a factor.

"I see many mothers who would like their daughters to be thinner," says Marjorie Laird, psychotherapist and director of the Freedom Program, an eating disorders outpatient program in Ontario, California. "The focus is on 'You can't eat that,' or

'Don't you think you're getting a little heavy?'"

Weight-obsessed moms are a national phenomenon. "I know moms who take their daughters to diet clinics when they are five or 10 pounds overweight," says Greenwich, Connecticut, psychologist Ann F. Caron, the author of *Don't Stop Loving Me: A Reassuring Guide for Mothers of Adolescent Daughters.* "When boys eat, we say, 'Isn't that wonderful,' but when girls eat, all too often we tend to say, 'Wait a minute—watch your weight!'"

Even girls who aren't overweight may get this message from their moms, according to a study of 2,000 girls ages 11 to 18 and 1,300 mothers conducted by Adam Drewnowski, a professor of public health at the University of Michigan in Ann Arbor. The study showed that one in three girls is on a diet, and a third of them with the encouragement of their mothers. Ironically, the girls in the study were of normal weight, so "clearly the need to diet was exaggerated," says Drewnowski.

And potentially dangerous as well. Early dieting can lead to stunted growth, delayed puberty, future health problems—such as osteoporosis—and a life-long bad body image, says Drewnowski.

> Daughters weigh their mothers' words heavily.

It can also be an entree to an eating disorder, which affects between five and 10 percent of American girls, according to the EDAP.

Often, as in Megan's case, the pressure to become thin begins at puberty, when it's perfectly natural for a girl to gain 30 pounds. "Moms and daughters have the perception that this weight gain means the daughter is becoming fat, even though it is completely normal and healthy," says Drewnowski.

Mom's Words Weigh Heavily

A comment from Mom about her weight can affect a girl even more so than one from a boy, girlfriend or even Dad. "Mom is a daughter's first role model, and the mother-daughter bond is incredibly strong," says Caron. "They are raised to look up to her, to want to be like her, to please her, so anything she says really goes to the heart."

Indeed, daughters weigh their mothers' words heavily. In a recent Heart, Lung and Blood Institute study of 2,379 girls 9 and 10 years old, researchers found that girls whose mothers tell them they are fat are more likely to lose weight and twice as likely to become chronic dieters.

This makes sense to Caron: "The more a mom bugs a girl to be thin, the greater the likelihood of the girl deciding that she will become so thin, her mom will never bug her again."

Of course, moms don't always use such blunt language to motivate a daughter to diet. In fact, girls are so sensitive to their mothers' opinions that all it takes is a word, a glance, even a facial expression.

"My mom tells me I'm beautiful, not to worry about how much I weigh," says 16-year-old Kristen Smith, who stands 5-feet 8-inches and is of average weight. "But sometimes, when I'm kind of chowing down, she does this thing where she blows her cheeks out, kind of like 'don't be a pig': It doesn't exactly hurt my feelings, but it sure makes me think twice about what I am eating." It also makes her doubt her mother when she says comforting things about her weight.

Other times, it's what a mom doesn't say or do that hits hard. Sandra Lowell remembers going on a diet when she was around 13: "I was a normal size, but I decided to go on a diet, and Mom said OK," she recalls. "I think I had hoped she would say, 'Honey, you don't need to'; but she didn't. I lost 15 pounds, but I was pretty thin to begin with and didn't need to."

Moms Really Mean Well

Mothers who encourage their daughters to diet do so with good intentions. They don't mean to be insensitive or heap on undue pressure—what they really want is for their daughters to be happy. "Mothers want their daughters to have people love and accept them," says Caron. "And girls who are overweight are often shunned."

Moms also want their daughters to look and feel beautiful. "In today's society, the message is that to be beautiful means to be thin, to wear a size two," Caron says. "Moms buy into that message and unconsciously impose it on their daughters."

> Mothers who encourage their daughters to diet do so with good intentions.

"I was completely shocked when my daughter and I were in the drugstore and she tossed a package of diet pills into our cart," says Janis Therman, whose daughter's action was an eye-opening experience for her. "I said, 'Vanessa! You don't need these!' And she replied, 'What do you mean, Mom? You're the one who's always telling me not to eat like a horse!' I had no idea I was making my daughter feel badly about herself!"

Moms who are overweight may project their body problems onto their daughters, seeing fat where there is none. Or an overweight mom may urge her daughter to diet to protect her from the pain she's known.

This was the signal Sandra's mom gave her. "My mom was 50 pounds overweight," she remembers. "She hated her body, and made comments about how disgusting it was. The subtext of everything she said and did was, 'Whatever you do, don't be like me.'"

Like Mother, Like Daughter

Daughters may also get the message to diet indirectly from their mothers through the mom's self-criticisms and/or food obsessions. "If a mom walks around saying she is fat, voicing disgust, saying she hates her thighs or is always dieting, constantly talking about fat and calories, the daughter can't help but pick up on that," says Rebecca Manley, founder and executive director of the Massachusetts Eating Disorder Association in Brookline.

"A daughter basically learns about the caring and nurturing of her body from her mother," adds Carolyn Costin, director of the Eating Disorders Center of California in Malibu and author of *Your Dieting Daughter.* "So how the mother not only cares for the daughter's body, but for her own body, has a huge influence on the girl."

> Daughters internalize not only their mothers' dieting habits, but also their bad body images.

This may explain why in Drewnowski's study, all of the girls who were dieting had mothers who were also on diets. Daughters internalize not only their mothers' dieting habits, but also their bad body images.

A mom who talks a good-eating game plan can't hide her own unhealthy food patterns. "I see a lot of mothers dieting, restricting food, compulsively exercising, who try to tell their daughters to eat breakfast as they grab a cup of coffee and run out the door," says Costin. "This 'do as I say, not as I do' won't work."

Breaking the Pattern

If you're feeling pressure from your mother to be thinner, talk to her about how you are feeling. "Most moms will appreciate your honesty," says Manley. Your mom may not even be aware she was being judgmental or critical, or that her words could wound so deeply. This gives her a chance to change.

Talking honesty and openly will also give you the opportunity to see if you have misinterpreted some of her comments or actions. Perhaps part of the pressure to be thin is coming from you or from friends. Together, you and your mom (along with input from your family physician) can determine if you really do need to lose weight and, if so, how your mother can provide you with positive support.

Talk to your mom about her dieting habits and body image, suggests Costin. Ask her how food and eating was handled when she was growing up. Ask how she feels about pressure from society and the media to be thin. The better you understand your mom, the more perspective you'll gain into her eating and dieting patterns. It may also be helpful to distance yourself from your mom's dieting patterns and food behavior—to recognize that you're not your mother's body.

For one young woman, Brittany Ellis, this realization was key to overcoming bulimia after she spent six years trying not to become an overweight yo-yo dieter like her mother. "As I grow up, I realize that I'm not my mother," says Brittany, now 22 and recovering from her eating disorder. "I'll always resemble her and have a bond with her, but I now know I don't have to embrace her misery or her patterns. I'm my own person."

Girls' Special Dieting Dilemma

Linda Ojeda

In the following article, Linda Ojeda explains why girls are more susceptible to weight gain than boys. Ojeda contends that girls' bodies are designed for motherhood, and a certain amount of fat is necessary to maintain reproductive functions, such as menstruation. Female sex hormones, estrogen and progesterone, not only hold on to fat, but also cause the body to produce more fat. These biological processes, combined with unhealthy eating and exercise habits, make it difficult for many girls to maintain a normal weight, which often leads to dieting. Ojeda is a lecturer and a certified nutritional consultant.

I don't know about you, but as I was growing up there were many things I didn't understand—and was afraid to ask about. Maybe that was more typical of my generation than yours. We didn't talk openly about things like sex, pregnancy, and contraception. In fact, we rarely even mentioned our periods to our best friends. Can you imagine that? The female body was a taboo topic. I'm so glad things have changed and girls are now free to discuss these subjects. The teenage years are scary enough. When you don't know what's going on and you don't feel comfortable asking, all sorts of strange thoughts go through your mind, exaggerating any problem.

Even though communication has improved over the years, there are some subjects that are not written about as much as others. This is true in the area of dieting and the female body. While dieting in general is a hot topic, the differences between males and females are often overlooked.

> Girls gain weight more easily than guys.

Female weight loss is affected by more variables than male weight loss. It is really true that girls gain weight more easily than guys, and shed pounds more slowly. It is also true that some girls have it easier than others, and even for the same individual, losing fat may be more difficult at certain times of the month than at others. Let's consider these points in more detail, one at a time.

Girls Are Born with More Fat than Guys

The female body is different from the male. My guess is you've already noticed! Our bodies are constructed to carry and feed an infant, regardless of whether or not we are having one. From the beginning of the child-bearing years (menarche) to their completion (menopause), our body's composition and our female hormones continuously prepare us to carry on life. This basic difference, as wonderful and miraculous as it is, makes it easier for us to put on weight and harder for us to lose it.

From the day a baby girl comes into the world, she is at a disadvantage in terms of fat. The female body has almost twice as much fat as the male. While guys carry around more muscle (which burns calories), girls store more fat (which doesn't burn calories). Muscle tissue burns five calories per pound more than fat tissue. This means that if you ate the same foods as your boyfriend or brother, and he stayed the same, you would gain weight. On the other hand, if you maintained your weight eating the same food, he would lose. Never diet with a guy friend. It's too depressing!

When girls exercise and increase their muscle mass, they too burn more calories, just like the guys. This doesn't mean the body becomes masculine—it can't, because female hormones prevent that. But it is a definite advantage for girls to build up their muscle and raise their metabolism. You will lose weight more quickly and you will be able to eat more.

Girls Make Fat Easily

The female body has a high percentage of slow-burning fat tissue. And, even though most of us are not thrilled with this fact, it helps us to understand why our bodies fight us when we try to diet. As I mentioned before, our extra fat is necessary to survival and our body hates to lose it. In fact, our fat is so linked to childbearing that when a female's body fat falls below 17% of her total weight, she will stop having periods and will no longer be able to carry a child. Our sex is designed for motherhood, whether we like it or not.

You probably know girls who stopped having periods when they got very skinny, or you may have friends who have not even started menstruating yet. Look at their bodies. You will see they don't have much body fat. When they put on some pounds, they will start or restart their cycle.

> Our extra fat is necessary to survival and our body hates to lose it.

Estrogen is the female hormone that directly affects shape and fat distribution. The more estrogen your body makes, the more "full-figured" you are. In other words, you have more fat on your hips, thighs, and breasts. Some people refer to this as an hourglass figure. The good news is, this look is supposedly coming back, and I personally know many guys like it. The bad news is, this shape makes it easier for you to gain weight and harder for you to lose it.

Let me tell you more about estrogen. As you probably know it is made in the ovaries. It is a hormone that loves to take the food you eat and turn it into fat. Remember, the female body is designed to keep fat on the body and it is estrogen's job to make sure this happens. So, if your body naturally makes more estrogen, your chances of being overweight are greater. But this is only part of the story. What you may not know is that estrogen is also manufactured from fat. Therefore, if you have more fat on your body, you are also going to *make* more estrogen.

> The more estrogen you have, the easier it is to store fat.

So, here's the picture. The more estrogen you have, the easier it is to store fat; the more fat you have, the more estrogen you make. You can see that once you start gaining weight, the body becomes a virtual fat-making machine.

Now you can see why it is harder for females who naturally make more estrogen to lose weight. Their bodies are working against them. While they struggle to lose fat, their bodies just love to make it. We often blame failure at dieting on our lack of will-power or self-control, when in fact it is our physiology. But don't take this knowledge and give up, thinking it's no use. You *can* lose the extra fat and you can keep it off. But you do have to work harder than a guy and harder than your friend who was born to be a stick.

Let me give you a few tips that are especially important if you have a full-figured body:

1. **Watch high fat foods,** because fatty foods are stored faster than any other kind.
2. **Eat more high fiber foods** (fruits, vegetables, whole grain breads, cereals, and pastas), because they help to lower estrogen levels in the body and assist in removing fat.
3. **Eat small meals more often,** since too much food at one time turns to fat.

4. **Watch salty foods,** because they retain water.
5. **Exercise regularly** to burn fat and build muscle.

Female Hormones and Cravings

A female's appetite appears to fluctuate with the ups and downs of her female hormones, estrogen and progesterone. Estrogen seems to reduce hunger while progesterone stimulates the appetite. After ovulation, which is half way through the menstrual cycle (for most girls this is two weeks after your period), estrogen levels fall and progesterone levels rise. When this happens, you may want to eat more than normal and you may find you crave particular foods like chocolate or chips.

How many of you have powerful cravings for candy, cookies, cheese puffs, or cake? I know there have been many days when I would make a special trip to the nearest bakery or finish off the stale potato chips because of this driving desire. I have one friend who told me that in one day she ate a pound of candy, a hot fudge sundae, and a chocolate mousse. I bet you can come up with a few stories of your own.

Food cravings can be caused by any number of things. It seems for many of us they get particularly strong right before our periods. Have you noticed this? If you haven't made that connection, the next time you want to eat everything in the kitchen, think about when your period is due. Chances are it's due in a few days.

Other things can also cause you to raid the refrigerator. Being overweight can itself result in binges, due to both psychological reasons (who cares? what's the use? food makes me feel good) and

> While [girls] struggle to lose fat, their bodies just love to make it.

physical or hormonal causes (blood sugar imbalances, insulin response). Still other possibilities include a lack of certain vitamins and minerals and poor eating habits (like too much sugar). Which of these apply to you? It could be more than one.

Female Hormones and Weight Loss

In the second half of the menstrual cycle, when progesterone is more dominant, there are other physiological changes that tend to make dieting harder or downright impossible. Some girls retain extra water so they feel bloated and fat, their fingers and stomach swell, and their breasts are painful or sensitive. Maybe you have noticed that the week before your period you often weigh several pounds more than you expect. Don't stress out. This is common. It just means you've gained water—not fat.

Retaining water is very discouraging to a dieter. You feel you've watched your calories all week and then you don't see the results on the scale. Even if you tell yourself it's probably water, psychologically you want to give up and give in. To avoid this, just before your period, when this is more likely to happen, relax on your diet. Don't expect to cut way back on your calories. Concentrate on simply maintaining your weight, and look forward to going back to your program in a few days.

> Retaining water is very discouraging to a dieter.

If you are prone to water retention there are several practical things you can do to keep it under control. Watch the amount of salty and sugary foods you eat, drink plenty of water (at least eight glasses a day), and eat several small meals rather than two or three large meals.

The Pill and Weight Gain

The oral contraceptive pill makes you retain water and also makes it easier for your body to convert food into fat. This means that if you are now maintaining your weight when eating 2,000 calories/day and you start taking the Pill, you will have to reduce your intake by 10% or 200 calories/day. There are other side effects of the Pill, too. If you feel any difference, tell your doctor. Since the Pill also affects your ability to absorb some nutrients, it would be smart to take a multiple vitamin/mineral tablet.

Inability to Handle Carbohydrates

Everyone would like to find a medical reason for being over-weight. When you go to the doctor for a checkup, you pray that she or he will discover some problem that can be fixed by taking a magic pill. Rarely do the tests find medical reasons for being overweight. (I know there are clinics that supply medications for weight loss, and I would like to warn you against them. The drugs prescribed have only temporary results and the people who take them do not lose weight any faster than others who do not. Unless there is a change in diet and lifestyle, no pill will have permanent results.)

There is a metabolic irregularity that has been found in some obese teenagers and adult women that causes them to store fat easily. Some females cannot process too many carbohydrates (breads, rice, beans, and pastas) at one time. While eating too much of any food causes weight gain, certain women cannot handle large amounts of starchy foods. Whether this condition causes obesity or obesity causes an intolerance to carbohydrates isn't clear. But if you feel you don't eat that much, this may be one reason you are not losing weight. Are you eating all your food at once? Try eating smaller meals, limit your starches to one per meal, and resist that second helping.

Tradition

This may or may not be a problem for you, at least not yet. In our societies, women are usually in charge of buying, preparing, and cooking the food. Being around food for a good part of the day and having to continually think about it is a real disadvantage to anyone who is susceptible to gaining weight. If you already find yourself in the kitchen baking cookies and trying out recipes on your family, be aware that tastes and nibbles have calories too and they quickly add up.

Chapter 2

Eating Disorders

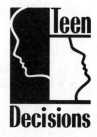

The Risks of Disordered Eating

Alison Bell

In the following article, Alison Bell contends that many teenage girls and young women dread getting fat and, in consequence, develop disordered eating habits—they constantly watch their weight and restrict calories. Many teens think that they are being healthy by regulating their diet and exercising frequently, but Bell maintains that most of them are not getting adequate calories, vitamins, and minerals to meet a teenager's dietary requirements. Moreover, she argues that strict diet and exercise regimens can lead to eating disorders such as anorexia (self-starvation) or bulimia (cycles of bingeing and purging). According to Bell, healthy eating means consuming at least fifteen hundred well-balanced calories a day of carbohydrates, protein, and fat. Bell is a contributor to *Teen Magazine*.

Millions of teenage girls have dangerous, way-out-of-whack eating behaviors, and they don't even know it.

From the minute she rolls out of bed, Amie Dahl, 19, has one thing on her mind: food. "I plan out all my meals in my head," says the hairstyling assistant from Arcadia, California. "I can't eat that, I can eat that." If she eats something she considers taboo—like an extra piece of bread (she limits herself to one slice a day) or some pasta (in general, she avoids carbohydrates)—"I feel terrible," Amie exclaims, "like I should go to the gym right now and burn it off!"

Sometimes she does. The StairMaster is Amie's current mode of maintaining her 5-foot 3-inch, 100-pound figure. When she was younger, she occasionally used laxatives to do the trick, but they made her dizzy. Now she just eats less and exercises more.

> Girls who restrict calories, constantly watch their weight and live in fear of getting fat are in the majority.

If you think there's nothing wrong with Amie's attitude toward eating, or even believe it's healthy, you're not alone. "Girls who restrict calories, constantly watch their weight and live in fear of getting fat are in the majority," says Boston College sociology professor Sharlene Hesse-Biber, Ph.D., author of *Am I Thin Enough Yet?*

The Big Deal on Your Body

If you don't think this majority has a problem, you're wrong. Healthy eating means consuming well-balanced, nutritious meals that add up to at least 1,500 calories a day and include adequate vitamins, minerals, protein, carbohydrates and, yes, fat. Healthy eating also requires an "everything in moderation" approach to treats—allowing yourself the occasional ice cream or potato chip indulgence. What's unhealthy is "leading a substandard, punishing life where how little you eat and weigh becomes the focus of your daily existence," says Carolyn Costin, Marriage, Family, and Child Counselor, director of the Malibu, California, Monte Nido Residential Treatment Center for eating disorders and author of *Your Dieting Daughter.* "It's like living in a calorie-counting prison."

This prison could lead to a bona fide eating disorder and eventually cause a host of life-threatening physical conditions. The less you eat, the more your body craves food—especially sugary stuff—to boost your sagging energy level. "Eventually you will binge," says Craig Johnson, Ph.D., director of the eating disorders program at Laureate Hospital in Tulsa, Oklahoma. Then you starve yourself to make up for the eating spree and could find yourself caught in a vicious starve-binge cycle.

Even if they don't develop bulimia or anorexia, girls with disordered eating still do major damage to their bodies. Calorie restriction and/or eliminating certain foods from your diet can make you sick. "Your body can go into a deprivation mode that can trigger nausea, fatigue, dizziness and irritability," says nutritionist Lisa Anes, B.A., a member of the American Dietetic Association and vice-president of the Health Economic Evaluations Database or H.E.E.D. Keep it up and food restriction can mess with your menstrual cycle, dry out your hair and skin and ultimately put you at risk for early onset of osteoporosis, a degenerative bone disease.

Since it's not easy to "rely" on willpower alone, many girls with disordered eating experiment with diuretics, laxatives, vomiting and diet supplements or pills. Even if you only use these things now and then, you're still playing with fire:

• Diuretics (or water pills) dehydrate the body, depleting it of sodium and potassium. In extreme cases, "this can cause irregularity of the heart, and you can go into shock and die," warns Sacker.

• Laxatives can cause heartburn, stomachaches and cramps, as well as possible permanent damage to your entire digestive system, says Anes. Because laxatives also function as diuretics, they can cause heart problems in some instances.

> Calorie restriction and/or eliminating certain foods from your diet can make you sick.

• Self-induced vomiting, even once in a while, can pop blood vessels in your face and swell up your neck glands, warns Anes.

Because your food isn't being digested properly, you may suffer stomachaches, constipation, diarrhea and reflex vomiting. Scarier still: There have been documented cases of people who made themselves vomit, ruptured their esophagus and died, Sacker says.

> If you don't eat enough while you're working out, your body feeds on its own muscles for energy.

• Diet pills are stimulants that can cause heart palpitations and jitters, especially if you build up a tolerance and end up overdosing, explains Sacker. They're also habit-forming once they wear off, you immediately become hungry and want to eat, so you reach for another pill to control your appetite.

• "Natural" diet supplements or "energy boosters" that contain ephedrine alkaloids, usually derived from the herb ma huang, are even more dangerous. The Food and Drug Administration reports that they've caused hundreds of medical problems, ranging from high blood pressure to heart attacks, strokes and death.

• Serious overexercising is also bad. When you overtrain, you tend to get more injuries. And if you don't eat enough while you're working out, your body feeds on its own muscles for energy. So instead of looking toned, you "can actually lose definition," says Anes.

The Big Deal on Your Mind

The physical problems disordered eating can cause are only half the picture. The emotional problems can be just as serious. A messed-up attitude toward food and body image is at the root of eating disorders and disordered eating alike. It makes some people "use" food as an artificial form of comfort or escape, much like a drug. (In some people, this "drowning your sorrows in food" can lead to obesity.) On the other side of the coin are those who restrict food because they feel that's the only part of their lives they can control. Either way, you wind up with a tortured preoccupation with food. Plus, the physical upheaval your body endures can make you moody, irritable and unable to concentrate. Worst of all, the more obsessed you become with eating (or not eating), the less you care about other things—school, sports, friends. "This can lead to depression and isolation," says Sacker. . . .

While some girls' disordered eating makes them withdraw, others bond over it. The most recent twist to this twisted mindset is groups of girls who get together for bingeing and purging en masse. They pig out then take turns going to the bathroom to vomit. This activity is "part competition to see who can exist on the fewest calories and part support group," says Anes—a sick way for girls to find acceptance and reinforce a behavior they otherwise might feel ashamed about.

They Don't Think They Have a Problem

As bizarre—and still relatively rare—as these splurge-and-purge sororities are, they point to the "safety in numbers" factor that perpetuates disordered eating. Lauren Richardson, 14, sees herself as pretty typical. "No one wants to be fat," asserts the Southern California teen. "If I got fat, I couldn't live with myself. I'd have no self-esteem." Yet despite being 5 feet 3 inches and only 107 pounds herself, Lauren believes she's got a weight problem. "People tell me I'm skinny, but I don't believe them," she says. After all, "everyone thinks they're overweight."

No, not everyone—but way too many adolescent girls do. In a study of 1,500 high school students, Del Mar, California, clinical psychologist Joni Johnston, Psy.D., found that 61 percent of girls

> 40 to 60 percent of all high school girls are on a diet.

sometimes felt fat. The same percentage said they felt guilty when they ate certain foods. Add to this the fact that some 40 to 60 percent of all high school girls are on a diet, and it makes for a very screwed-up picture.

One reason Lauren doesn't think she has a problem is because so many of her friends share the same attitude. "We live in a society where it's the standard for a teenager to worry excessively about her body and gaining weight," says Hesse-Biber. "This aberrant behavior has become the norm."

Experts point to the media for feeding teens' body obsessions.

Sara Johnson, 17, a recovering anorexic and bulimic from Monticello, Minnesota, who starved herself down from 136 to 92 pounds and existed on 212 calories of pretzels she ate and threw up—every day, was horrified to learn that she was a "role model." When a girl asked Sara how to make yourself vomit so she could do it too, "I blew up," recalls Sara. "I told her, 'You think I enjoy it? I hate being like this!'"

The Media's Influence

Experts point to the media for feeding teens' body obsessions, since they bombard audiences with a steady stream of skinny actresses and models. "Maybe only 5 percent of the population is 6 feet tall and weighs 109 pounds, but that is the artificial image girls are trying to live up to," says Susan Mackey, Ph.D., a clinical psychologist in Evanston, Illinois. When a girl does lose weight, she receives positive reinforcement from her peers who have also bought into the "thin is in" message, perpetuating her disordered eating.

But the media aren't the only culprits. Sadly, sometimes the people you love, trust and turn to for guidance inadvertently encourage disordered eating. Consider the feedback some girls get from their families. "My mother always told me, 'Don't eat so much,'" Amie says. "Even now, she says things like, 'You've got a belly.' That makes me feel gross."

Even if your mom doesn't rag on you about your weight, you can still follow her disordered eating lead. "Girls may pick up on their mothers' own unhealthy eating habits, even if they try to hide them," says Johnston, who is also the author of *Appearance Obsession.* Frances Berg, author of *Afraid to Eat: Children and Teens in Weight Crisis,* agrees: "Parents' dieting and fussing about weight sends destructive messages to kids."

Then there are the girls who go into athletics for all the right, healthy reasons and wind up on a track toward disordered eating. In such sports as gymnastics, diving and ice-skating, coaches may pressure girls to lose that extra 5 pounds for a better performance or look—which girls may misinterpret as an order to starve themselves, says Sacker.

> Parents' dieting and fussing about weight sends destructive messages to kids.

Whatever leads girls to fall into a pattern of disordered eating, they ultimately find themselves on a physical and emotional treadmill they don't know how to turn off. "It's exhausting to keep up my guard [against food] all the time," says Amie. "I wish I could just let it down."

Getting Your Life Back

Amie can let her guard down and start a healthy relationship with food—and if you recognize yourself in this story, so can you. Here's how:

• Don't believe the hype. While skinny images are all over advertising and the media, it's quite possible the real people behind those images are dealing with problems. Just think of all the celebs who've 'fessed up to dealing with eating disorders. "We live in a weight-obsessed culture, but you don't have to be brainwashed by it," says Johnston.

• Challenge your assumptions. Are you really going to get "fat" if you eat that extra cookie? Are all your friends honestly skinnier than you? Is being thin worth it if you have to worry about your weight all the time, not eat when you're hungry and engage in risky behavior like vomiting, using laxatives or taking over-the-counter diet pills?

• Change your language. Stop saying you're fat when you aren't. Call friends on the word when they use it loosely. This will make you even more aware of the fallacy of some of your own thinking.

• Figure out if something deeper is fueling your food issues, recommends Johnston. Worrying about your weight may mask other problems, such as unhappiness at home or at school.

• Channel your energies into sports, art, drama—any positive activity or pursuit that makes you feel good about yourself. The more energy you put toward other areas of your life, the less you'll expend obsessing over your weight, says Costin.

• Follow your body's natural needs. Eat when you feel hungry, as long as the food is nutritious, and stop when you are full. Realize that restricting certain food groups, like carbohydrates, is unnecessary and unhealthy unless you have a food allergy.

• Seek help if you think you need it. "Talk to a parent, adult friend or school counselor," says Johnston. If necessary, they can refer you to an expert in the field of eating disorders.

Elizabeth got help, and it's the best thing she ever did. Last year she was on her way to anorexia when her mother intervened and got her into counseling. "It could have been worse," says Elizabeth, whose life and weight are back on track, "a lot, lot worse."

Living with Anorexia

BriAnne Dopart

In the following article, twenty-year-old BriAnne Dopart describes her experience with anorexia in several fictional diary entries. Anorexia is a serious eating disorder in which people view themselves as being heavier than they actually are. Many anorexics use diet pills to control their appetites and laxatives to purge their bodies of food. Most anorexics refuse to eat enough calories to maintain health, and many exercise obsessively. In her story, BriAnne describes some of the physical effects of anorexia, such as bone damage from lack of calcium and yellow teeth. Other effects of anorexia are anemia (lack of iron), depression, and even death from starvation. If you or someone you know shows signs of anorexia, seek help immediately.

October 15, 1994
Dear BriAnne,

I'm writing to you because I feel like I'm alone and if anyone will know how I feel, it'll be you.

I just started the eighth grade. I have braces and I think I'm too fat to fit in any of the "trendy" clothes. My best friend has a crush on this guy, and I think he likes her back. Soon they'll be dating and then it'll be just me, walking home from school alone.

Excerpted from "Letters from Within: Looking Back at Living with Eating Disorders," by BriAnne Dopart, *Teen Voices*, Winter 2001. Copyright © 2001 by *Teen Voices*. Reprinted with permission.

I don't have many friends. My friends from sixth grade don't talk to me anymore. My friends all have boyfriends now.

I don't like to talk to the boys in my school because they probably think I'm ugly and don't want to talk to me. I don't want to talk to the girls because all they talk about is which boys they like and what they're going to wear tomorrow.

I'm in the "smart" English class now but my writing is still terrible. All of the other kids in that class know all these words I don't know. And every week Mrs. K picks an essay she thinks is the best and she reads it out loud. She hates my writing and gives me Cs on everything. She'll never pick one of mine.

I'm so tired of school, BriAnne. I'm tired of not being pretty like the other girls. I'm tired of no boys liking me. I'm tired of not being as cool or as smart or as whatever as the other kids. Something needs to change.

At home, Mom and Dad aren't much help. Since Scott's been dead they've been lost in their sadness. I know they are trying to pay attention to me but I feel like they care about him more now that he's dead, than they do for me alive. Maybe if I die, they'll love me more too.

I miss my brother, BriAnne. I miss my friends from sixth grade. I miss my old family. Really, I just want to go away.

I started this new diet on my thirteenth birthday. I don't really eat anything now but no one notices. My doctor told me it would just slow down my metabolism or something and make me fatter in the end. She said it would ruin my bones and my stomach and my hair and my teeth, but really, really, I'm ready to try anything. I'd do anything to just shrink away, BriAnne. I'd do anything to just disappear.

—Your 13-year-old self

April 16, 1998
Dear BriAnne,

I've been thinking forever about which words I could write to you to make you stop doing what you are about to do.

You're on a diet now, but soon it will be anorexia. When the anorexia doesn't work well enough, you'll try bulimia. By the time you are 17 you will be so skinny that your boyfriend will stop hugging you because he says the boniness makes him sick.

What Is Anorexia Nervosa?

Anorexia nervosa is characterized as a disorder in which people refuse to maintain a minimally normal weight, have an intense fear of gaining weight, and often misinterpret their body shape. For example, it is not uncommon for a woman suffering from anorexia to weigh only 15 percent of her normal body weight and still think she looks fat. Individuals who are plagued by anorexia are usually persistent in their pursuit for thinness. They usually possess characteristics of a perfectionist and are rather high functioning. Their pursuit to thinness often leads to starvation and this pursuit can lead to death.

Anorexia is an eating disorder that is more typical in women than in men and can come about at any age. But studies show that the onset typically happens in adolescence. However, in my practice, I have seen girls as young as age nine diagnosed with anorexia.

Shari Neufeld, Teen.com, January 2, 2001.

Anorexia takes hold of your brain, BriAnne. You'll think you're taking control but really it's taking control of you. Soon you'll lie and say anything to avoid eating. Soon you'll skip anything: a dance, a date, a trip to the movies with friends—just to avoid having to be around food.

Your parents will notice, but not the way you want them to. They won't understand that you're not in control anymore and they'll think you're doing it on purpose. And starving won't make them miss your brother any less, or make your pain go away either.

Your friends won't know what to do. Only your best friend Sumitra will stick around. One night she'll drop by around dinnertime to say hello, but the anorexia will have such a hold on you that you'll tell her to go home because you need to eat alone. She won't know what a good friend should do. She will just say, "O.K., I'll see you later," and she'll drive away and never mention it again.

You'll be so afraid to eat you won't do anything. You won't go with your friends to the mall because you won't want to have to walk by the food court. You'll cut your dates short with your boyfriend because eating your 10 P.M. meal of carrots is more important to you than finishing the video, the coffee, or the conversation.

> I'm tired of not being as cool or as smart or as whatever as the other kids.

One day, you'll be in a dressing room with your mother and you'll take off your shirt and she'll see how your ribs poke out from under your skin and she'll start crying. She'll beg you to stop killing yourself with starvation but by then you'll be too sick to care.

You'll get counseling, but you won't think you need it. Your therapist will tell you that you are destroying yourself and you won't believe her. Your hair will fall out, leaving a pile of blond strands in the drain after every shower. Your eyes will have dark-blue circles underneath them. Your collarbone will poke out of your skin. You'll stop getting your period. You'll start fainting when it's too hot out. But every day you'll look in the mirror and think, *Just a few more pounds to go.*

Soon you won't leave your house. Sometimes Sumitra will visit—but not as often as she used to. Your boyfriend will start seeing other people. You won't care. You'll weigh yourself every morning, every night, and every afternoon. The bathroom scale will be your new best friend. Soon even your poems will be about calories and pounds.

—Your 17-year-old self

June 16, 2001

Dear BriAnne,

I'm 19 now, BriAnne. This year I broke my ribs three times. I got an X-ray and the doctor told me that my bones were breaking easily because I deprived them of calcium for so long.

I've got stretch marks running up and down my legs and stomach because of how fast I lost weight. My teeth are yellowed because I was under-nourished for so long.

> I'd do anything to just shrink away.

I've got an ulcer now too. And my esophagus doesn't work right, so I throw up more often than normal, and my chest burns a lot. I can't eat oranges because they burn my esophagus. It's the same with tomatoes or spicy foods. My stomach forgot how to break down milk so I can't have ice cream anymore, not even just a little.

I have to take pills every day to keep my esophagus working right. I take pills every day to try to fix all the damage I did to my bones. I take iron pills to keep from becoming anemic again. Because starving prevents your brain from making serotonin [a chemical messenger that regulates emotion], I have to take pills every day to make more of it, so that I can try to be happy again.

I have to take so many pills that when somebody new comes over and sees my pill case in the bathroom, they think I have some horrible disease. And I do, BriAnne, I have anorexia-bulimia nervosa.

—Your 19-year-old-self

August 20, 2001

Dear BriAnne,

Please talk to someone. Talk to a relative, a teacher, or a mentor you can trust. Tell them how alone you feel. Tell them how you want to disappear. Tell them how you feel about your body and that starving or throwing up seems to be the answer.

More importantly than anything, try to tell your parents how you see them, how you feel, and what you think you need. If you can't say it out loud then try writing a letter to them. It's so important that they know.

And please, BriAnne, remember that you are so much more than you think you are. Inside of you right now is a talented, intelligent, loving young woman. You deserve the chance to become her.

So feed her. Take care of her. Let yourself grow into her. Let her grow into you.

—Your 20-year-old-self

Bulimia Causes Serious Health Problems

Mike Hardcastle

In the following article, a teenager asks for advice on identifying and treating bulimia. Bulimia is an eating disorder that is characterized by cycles of binge eating (eating large quantities of food in a sitting) and purging (eliminating the food by vomiting or using laxatives). Mike Hardcastle, an advice columnist for teenagers at the website About.com, contends that most anorexics and bulimics are in denial about the damage they are doing to their bodies. He asserts that eating disorders are often an effort to control some part of what the bulimic sees as an out-of-control life. He maintains that bulimia is a serious condition that requires professional help.

I am a little worried about my weight. What I need to know is how to tell if I have bulimia and if there is a way to treat it myself without my family knowing.

B ulimia nervosa and and anorexia nervosa are closely related disorders. Although both are commonly known as "eating disorders," they're actually classified as a "emotional disorders." Studies show that these disorders are rarely triggered by a real need to lose weight, but are actually extreme reactions to "out of control" family or social situations. The main difference between anorexia and bulimia is simple; anorexics starve themselves, bulimics binge and purge.

Identifying Bulimia

Since you asked about bulimia, let's look at the most obvious features of this disorder. Things to look for when identifying bulimia are:

1. Periods of withholding food (starvation) followed by eating binges ("pig outs").
2. Eating binges in response to a stressful or disappointing event.
3. Binge eating followed by purging, either by induced vomiting, or regular use of laxatives.
4. Guilt and "self punishment" (in the form of starvation) after a binge.

Since bulimics are rarely obese to begin with, the initial weight loss often goes unnoticed by others. But bulimics do lose weight, and like anorexics, they lose it quickly and dangerously. The rapid weight loss associated with both the disorders can cause electrolyte depletion, jaundice, low blood pressure, vitamin deficiency, and irregular menstruation in girls. Bulimics often have: dry skin, white heads, yellow eyes, bad breath, weak or brittle nails and hair, cold hands and feet, rotten teeth or teeth with little or no enamel (caused by vomiting), problems controlling bowel movements and urination (if laxatives are used).

> [Eating] disorders are rarely triggered by a real need to lose weight.

The starvation of both bulimia and anorexia put tremendous strain on the body's internal organs. An estimated 2–5% of cases, the disorders cause the body to shut down completely resulting in death. Both disorders are more common in girls than in boys, but they do occur in both sexes. As stated earlier, these disorders are emotional disorders and are thought to be passive aggressive attempts to reclaim a sense of control over one's life.

The Costs of Bulimia

Teens with bulimia nervosa maintain a normal body weight. But sneaky trips to the bathroom after meals and secret binges indicate serious problems. The bulimic gets stuck in a binge and purge cycle. Vomiting doesn't just get rid of unwanted calories; it gives a deep sense of relief. Like any other drug, it makes you temporarily feel better. A bulimic may steal money just to support her habit, which can cost as much as $50 a day. Extreme binges? The equivalent of 210 brownies, or 20,000 calories. Average binges are around 3,400 calories, about an entire pecan pie.

Bulimia goes untreated far longer than anorexia because a person with bulimia keeps it secret. The anorexic denies there is anything wrong, but the bulimic hides in shame.

Sophia Schweitzer, Teenwire.com, February 21, 2001.

Bulimia is twofold; it's a course of action and an emotional state. It is impossible to properly diagnose yourself. However, bulimics and anorexics share certain traits (or causes). These conditions characteristically affect girls of middle and upper middle-class families. They usually first appear between the ages of 10 and 20, although both conditions can persist well into adulthood. Bulimics and anorexics are usually good students who obey the rules and are generally cooperative and complacent. These generalizations are based on controlled studies; as with any "rule" there are exceptions (as noted above, males can suffer from these disorders).

Get Professional Help

As to treatment, you must get professional help. You do not need to tell your family until you're ready to, but you must tell somebody. You can get treatment in support groups, free clinics and crisis lines. You can even find help online, in virtual support groups, chat sessions and bulletin boards. There are lots of places you can turn to for help while still remaining anonymous. The only reason you may have to tell your parents is if you seek medical treatment that you need to pay for or for which you need to file an insurance claim. If you want to avoid this, your best bet is a free clinic. Most people find that once they start treatment they want to share their stories with others. If and when you reach this point, it would be a very good idea to tell your family and loved ones what you are going through so they can better support your recovery.

> Bulimics and anorexics are usually good students who obey the rules.

At the very least, you must stop the cycle of starvation, binging and purging. If you can't go to the doctor for help in doing this, you must find a support group. You must eat normally and gain weight. It is best if you get medical attention as soon as possible since there are medications that can help you in your recovery. Bulimia is a mental disorder that affects you physically; for this reason a doctor must be involved in any recovery effort. Bulimia is not like a cold; you can not take care of it yourself. You need help, support and medical attention. Depending on the degree of your bulimia, it could be dangerous to rapidly put on the weight you lost. If you do attempt to treat yourself there will likely come a time when you will need and want outside help. Don't be afraid to reach out to those closest to you since they are most likely to notice if you start to slip or if the bulimic behavior returns.

Denial

A big part of both bulimia and anorexia is denial. People who suffer from these disorders are in denial about what they're doing to their bodies, and what is going on in their lives. Since this type of emotional disorder is brought on by a desire to control some part of a seemingly out of control life, it is very easy for sufferers to feel vindicated by what they're doing to their bodies. If you suspect you are bulimic, I strongly urge you to get a medical opinion. Go to a free clinic, go to a family doctor, see your school nurse, see somebody in the medical profession and find a reliable support system that includes a psychiatrist or therapist. You cannot get over bulimia alone.

Boys and Eating Disorders

John DiConsiglio

According to John DiConsiglio in the following article, eating disorders affect more than one million males in the United States. This figure may be conservative due to the fact that many men and boys with eating disorders see anorexia and bulimia as female problems and fail to seek help. DiConsiglio contends that most boys and men with eating disorders are athletes trying to control their weight for competition. For example, wrestlers may adopt extreme diet and exercise practices to lose weight for a match. He suggests that if you or someone you know exhibits dangerous eating and exercise habits, seek help immediately. DiConsiglio is a contributor to *Scholastic Choices*, a monthly magazine that focuses on topics relevant to today's teens.

M ike thought eating disorders were just a girls' problem— until he began wasting away.

For the life of him, Mike Rogerson couldn't figure out why he was being called down to the library in the middle of the school day. The 15-year-old high school sophomore from Davenport, Florida, was certain that he had no overdue books. What could be important enough to drag him out of class?

Mike was really astonished when he swung open the library doors. Seated around a table were his best friend, Tom Wilson, and three of his favorite teachers. At first, Mike thought he was in trouble—or that something had happened to his family. But his English teacher put a hand on Mike's shoulder and said, "Mike, something is going on with you. I think you have an eating disorder. And you're not leaving this library until you get help."

"Are you crazy!" Mike said. "Girls get eating disorders. Not guys." But Mike was dead wrong. In the space of a month, he'd lost more than 50 pounds from his 6-foot 5-inch frame—dropping from 214 pounds to 160. Like millions of young people, Mike was suffering from an eating disorder. And, like many others, Mike never imagined that diseases like anorexia and bulimia could strike a male.

It's true that most people with eating disorders are female, but males also suffer. According to a new study, one in six eating-disorder victims are men or boys,

> Many men deny that they have an eating disorder.

totaling more than 1 million males in the U.S. Most, experts say, are athletes struggling to control their weight for competition.

"Eating disorders in men aren't well understood. And to an extent, they aren't taken very seriously," says Vivian Hanson Meehan, R.N., founder of the National Association of Anorexia Nervosa and Associated Disorders (ANAD).

"Many men deny they have an eating disorder," she says. "It's hard to get them to accept help."

Denying the Problem

That day in the library, Mike wasn't looking for help, though his friend and teachers knew he had a serious problem. He was exercising incessantly—running three miles a day with weighted garbage bags taped beneath sweatpants. He was throwing away his lunch every day.

"I insisted there was nothing wrong with me," says Mike, now 20. "I was just dropping a few pounds for wrestling. I told them I'd be over it in a week or two."

Sadly, Mike was wrong. He still hasn't beaten his eating disorder—though he has been under a psychotherapist's and medical doctor's care for more than five years. His weight has dropped to as low as 127 pounds, but when he looks in the mirror, he sees an obese monster. He had originally suffered from bulimia—where he binged on massive amounts of food and then "purged" by throwing up or using laxatives and diuretics. Now he is anorexic—he starves himself, fasting for as long as a month at a time.

> A certain amount of everyone's body weight has to be fat.

His inability to eat has caused massive internal damage. A certain amount of everyone's body weight has to be fat. The kidneys, liver, and other organs need fat to function. Mike's eating disorder has left his kidneys and liver badly damaged. His bulimia has deprived his body of potassium, which can lead to heart failure—the prime cause of death related to eating disorders. Indeed, a lack of fat and potassium has caused Mike's heart to shrink.

Feeling Worthless

Mike thinks his problem began because of a bad relationship with his father. "He was verbally abusive toward me," he says. "He's a harsh guy. He was always calling me fat and lazy. He would tell me I'd never amount to much in life."

Mike was an A student, but felt worthless. To please his dad, he went out for the wrestling team. "I'm tall, so I weighed over 200 pounds," Mike says. "But all the other guys in my weight class were made of muscle. I knew I couldn't compete with them." Mike decided he had to drop enough weight to qualify for a lighter weight class.

He started an intense workout regime. But when he failed to

lose enough weight, he turned to a different solution. He began bingeing and purging. He ate enormous quantities of food, downing hamburger after hamburger. Then, when he was alone, Mike forced himself to vomit.

"I thought it was just temporary, until I made the weight," Mike says. "But when I made the weight, I was so weak that I couldn't wrestle."

> His constant forced vomiting had torn the lining of his stomach.

That's when his friends and teachers cornered Mike in the library. Then, a few days later, in the middle of history class, Mike began vomiting blood. It turns out that his constant forced vomiting had torn the lining of his stomach. His mom rushed him to a doctor, who delivered sobering news.

"He told me that what I was doing would eventually kill me," Mike says.

Tough Road Back

Mike agreed to get help. Eating disorders are curable, and most cases are not as severe as Mike's. The most successful treatment, experts say, combines therapy to heal the psychological scars, and food reeducation to teach sufferers how to eat healthy again. Mike has had some victories, but each time he has fallen back into defeat. While he had his weight up to nearly 160, after a recent relapse he was back to 137.

The worst part, he says, is the loneliness. "No one understands this," he says. "Every day, from the moment I wake up to the time I go to bed, I think about this. This isn't a normal life."

But Mike hasn't given up hope. "Right now, I'm focusing on staying alive," he says. "And every day that I'm still here gives me another day to fight."

Eating Disorders: The Facts

• How many people have eating disorders? Experts estimate that 8 million Americans—males and females combined—suffer from eating disorders. Ninety percent of them developed the disease before age 20. One study found that 11 percent of high school seniors suffer from an eating disorder.

• What causes eating disorders? There's no single cause, though eating disorders are almost always a symptom of some emotional issue. Many people say the media contribute to the problem by bombarding teens with images of wispy thin models and supercut studs.

• What is anorexia? Starving yourself to take off weight, and thinking you're fat even though you're not.

• What is bulimia? Eating lots of food in one sitting, and then purging the food (usually by vomiting or using laxatives).

• How do eating disorders hurt your health? Anorexics develop all the symptoms of malnutrition, including heart, kidney, and liver damage. Bulimics often develop ulcers, irregular heartbeats, and rotten teeth (from acid in the vomit). . . .

Are You at Risk?

Below are some warning signs of an unhealthy relationship with food. Read the list and check any item that describes you. If you check one or more, you may have a problem—but don't panic. Discuss your concerns with a parent school counselor or doctor.

• You weigh yourself frequently and feel fat even when the mirror shows you aren't.

• You sneak food or lie about your eating habits.

• You don't like to eat in front of other people and skip social events because you know food will be served.

• You starve yourself for a day, then overeat and hate yourself for it.

• You occasionally purge by vomiting or using laxatives, or you exercise for hours when it's not part of supervised athlete training.

Chapter 3

How to Lose Weight Healthfully

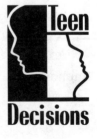

Dieting Basics

Nutricise

In the following article, Nutricise, a comprehensive on-line resource for nutrition and fitness information, provides an overview of teenagers and dieting. The site explains that some teens diet to get in shape for sports while others do so because they think that they should be thin like fashion models. If you feel that you need to lose weight, Nutricise suggests that rather than dieting, you should eat balanced meals in accordance with the U.S. Department of Agriculture's (USDA) Food Guide Pyramid and get plenty of vigorous exercise.

If you watch television, see movies, read newspapers or flip through magazines, you've probably noticed that diets are everywhere. High-protein diets. Low-fat diets. All-vegetable diets. No-pasta diets. But with all the focus on dieting, how do you figure out what's healthy and what isn't? Many teens feel pressured to lose weight and try different types of diets, but if you really need to lose weight, improving your eating habits and exercising will help you more than any diet. Here are the basics of dieting:

People diet for many reasons. Some teens weigh too much and need to pay closer attention to their eating and exercise habits. Some teens play sports and want to be in top physical condition. Other teens may feel they would look and feel better if they lost a few pounds.

Some teens may diet because they think they are "supposed" to look a certain way. Models and actresses are thin, and many of today's fashions are modeled by very thin people. But the model-thin style is an unrealistic look for most people. By around ages 12 or 13, most teen girls go through body changes that are natural and necessary: their hips broaden, their breasts develop and suddenly the way they look may not match girls in television or magazine ads.

> Some teens may diet because they think they are "supposed" to look a certain way.

Can Diets Be Unhealthy?

Any diet that suggests you eat fewer calories than you need to get through the day (such as an 800 calories-a-day diet) is dangerous. Diets that don't allow any fat can also be bad for you. You should have a certain amount of fat in your diet, between 20 and 25 percent of your total calories. Although a low-fat diet may be okay, don't go completely fat-free.

Don't fall for diets that restrict certain food groups, either. A diet that says "no" to breads or pastas or allows you to eat only fruit is unhealthy. You won't get the vitamins and minerals you need and although you may lose weight, you'll probably gain it back as soon as you start eating in your usual way.

Some teens start dieting because they think all the problems in their lives are weight-related. Or some teens have an area of their lives that they can't control—an alcoholic parent, for example—so they focus excessively on something they can control—their exercise and food. Once these teens start losing weight, they may get lots of praise and compliments from friends and family, which makes them feel good. But they will eventually reach a weight plateau, and they won't lose as much weight as before because their body is trying to maintain a healthy weight. They may also find they aren't any happier, but they still keep their main focus on their weight.

Some teens may find it hard to control their eating, so they control it for a little while, but then eat tons of food. Feeling guilty about the binge, they use laxatives or vomit. Both of these problems are eating disorders, which are harmful to a person's health. A teen with an eating disorder needs medical treatment right away.

So How Can I Lose Weight Safely?

Dieting usually means severely restricting calories or certain food groups. When you're a teen, dieting can be dangerous because you may not get the right kind and right amount of nutrients, which can lead to poor growth and other health problems. In other words, by not eating right your height could even fall short!

But eating healthy meals and snacks and getting a reasonable amount of exercise may help you lose weight and develop properly at the same time. For a lot of teens, just being more active might help you lose weight without even changing what you eat! So get moving—whether you're involved in sports or you just take a walk or a bike ride several days a week, exercise really helps.

The most important thing to remember when you are dieting is to eat a wide variety of food to ensure that you're meeting

> Don't fall for diets that restrict certain food groups.

your body's needs. Try to cut back on high-fat meats (like burgers and hot dogs), eat more fruits and vegetables and drink more water instead of sugary drinks like sports drinks or sodas.

For many teens, just exercising more and following a healthy diet (use the Food Guide Pyramid) can help you stay in shape and achieve a healthy weight. But if you are concerned about your body's size or think you need to lose weight, talk with a medical professional first—a doctor or dietitian may even reassure you that you are at a healthy weight. If you are overweight, the doctor can help you determine the best way to reach a healthy weight.

Great Ways to Find Great Health

Here are some tips to help you change your health habits:

- Exercise!
- Drink milk, including fat-free or low-fat milk. Many teens mistakenly think that milk has more calories than other drinks, such as soda. But a glass of skim milk has only 80

USDA Food Guide Pyramid

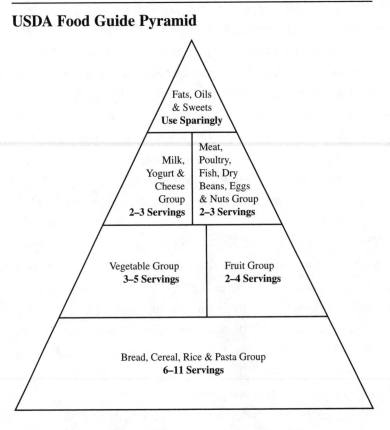

U.S. Department of Agriculture and U.S. Department of Health and Human Services, Food Guide Pyramid.

calories as well as protein and calcium. Soda has 120 calories of sugar and no other nutrients.

- Eat a variety of foods, including plenty of fruits and vegetables.
- Drink plenty of water.
- Eat lean, high-protein foods, like lean meat, chicken, fish or beans.
- Eat grains, which provide fiber, B vitamins and iron.
- Eat breakfast. Studies show that people who eat breakfast do better in school, and tend to eat less throughout the day.
- Watch out for excessive caffeine—it doesn't help you lose weight and can cause dehydration.
- Stay away from fad diets—even if you lose five pounds, you'll just gain it back when you go back to your usual way of eating.
- Don't take diet pills, even ones you get over the counter, unless prescribed by your doctor or dietitian.
- Don't get into an "I don't eat that" way of thinking. If you eliminate entire food groups, you may miss out on important nutrients.
- If you choose to become a vegetarian, talk to your doctor or dietitian about how to make good, nutritious vegetarian choices.

Dieting Danger Signs

How do you know if your diet or a friend's diet is out of control? If you or a friend does any of the following things, talk to a doctor:

- Continues to diet, even if not overweight
- Has physical changes, such as weakness, headaches or dizziness
- Withdraws from family and friends
- Performs poorly in school
- Eats in secret

- Thinks about food all the time
- Restricts activities because of food or compulsive exercise
- Fears food
- Wears baggy clothes to hide thinness
- Uses laxatives or vomits

Dieting and weight control can consume your life. By accepting your body and making healthy choices, you'll keep your weight under control and enjoy life.

Deciding to Go on a Diet

Ruth Papazian

In the following article, Ruth Papazian contends that many teenagers are pressured by their family or friends to be very thin, and some teenagers diet even though they are not overweight. Teens with legitimate weight concerns may adopt dangerous weight loss methods, such as fad dieting, taking weight loss pills, or vomiting. These habits can be hazardous to teens' health because limiting food intake can deprive the body of nutrients that are essential to growth and development. Moreover, unhealthy eating habits can turn into life-threatening eating disorders such as anorexia nervosa and bulimia nervosa. If you think you may need to lose weight, consult your doctor to devise a healthy, safe, and effective eating and exercise plan. Papazian is a freelance writer who specializes in health and medicine.

W hat do the hula hoop, "high-protein diets," and wearing your clothes backwards have in common? They are all fads. Fads come and go, but when it comes to fad diets, the health effects can be permanent—especially for teenagers.

Not all teens who go on diets need to lose weight. Pressure

From "On the Teen Scene: Should You Go on a Diet?" by Ruth Papazian, *FDA Consumer Magazine*, September 1993.

from friends—and sometimes parents—to be very slim may create a distorted body image. Having a distorted body image is like looking into a funhouse mirror: You see yourself as fatter than you are.

A national survey of 11,631 high school students conducted by the national Centers for Disease Control and Prevention found that more than a third of the girls considered themselves overweight, compared with fewer than 15 percent of the boys. More than 43 percent of the girls reported that they were on a diet—and a quarter of these dieters didn't think they were overweight. The survey found that the most common dieting methods used were skipping meals, taking diet pills, and inducing vomiting after eating.

"The teenage years are a period of rapid growth and development," points out Ronald Kleinman, M.D., chief of the Pediatric Gastrointestinal and Nutrition Unit of Massachusetts General Hospital in Boston. He explains that fad dieting can keep teenagers from getting the calories and nutrients they need to grow properly and that dieting can retard growth. Stringent dieting may cause girls to stop menstruating, and will prevent boys from developing muscles, he says. If the diet doesn't provide enough calcium, phosphorus and vitamin D, bones may not lay down enough calcium. This may increase the risk of osteoporosis later in life, although more studies are needed to confirm this.

> Not all teens who go on diets need to lose weight.

Instead of dieting because "everyone" is doing it or because you are not as thin as you want to be, first find out from a doctor or nutritionist whether you are carrying too much body fat for your age and height.

What If You Need to Lose Weight?

The flip side to feeling pressured to be thin is having legitimate concerns about [being] overweight that adults dismiss by saying, "It's just baby fat" or "You'll grow into your weight." Most girls reach almost their full height once they start to menstruate, notes Kleinman. Although boys usually don't stop growing until age 18, data from a study suggest that adolescent obesity can carry serious life-long health consequences for them.

> The longer in adolescence you remain overweight, the greater the likelihood that the problem will persist into adulthood.

The study, which followed the medical histories of 508 people from childhood to age 70, found that men who had been overweight teenagers were more likely to develop colon cancer and to suffer fatal heart attacks and strokes than their thinner classmates. Women who had been overweight teens had an increased tendency to develop clogged arteries (atherosclerosis) and arthritis. By age 70, these problems made it difficult for them to walk more than a quarter mile, lift heavy objects, or climb stairs.

While this study linked adolescent obesity to health problems decades down the road, some adverse effects show up much earlier. Sometimes teens develop high blood pressure, elevated cholesterol, and conditions that often precede diabetes. Also, as Kleinman points out, "The longer in adolescence you remain overweight, the greater the likelihood that the problem will persist into adulthood."

The Wrong Way to Lose Weight

As with most everything else, there's a right way and a wrong way to lose weight. The wrong way is to skip meals, resolve to eat nothing but diet bread and water, take diet pills, or make yourself vomit. You may make it through the end of the week and maybe even lose a pound or two, but you're unlikely to keep the weight off for more than a few months—if that. And inducing vomiting can lead to an eating disorder called bulimia, which can result in serious health problems.

"The more you deprive yourself of the foods you love, the more you will crave those foods. Inevitably, you'll break down and binge," says Jo Ann Hattner, a clinical dietitian at Packard Children's Hospital in Palo Alto, California. Then you'll not only gain those pounds back, you'll likely add a couple more.

Experts call this cycle of weight loss and weight gain "yo-yo" dieting. Obesity researchers believe that truly overweight people should continue to try to control their weight because studies are inconclusive on whether weight cycling is harmful, according to the National Institute of Diabetes and Digestive and Kidney Diseases. In contrast, the health risks from being overweight are well-known. Although the yo-yo effect may not hurt future weight-loss efforts, you need to make lifelong changes in eating behavior, diet, and physical activity.

> Rapid weight loss from very-low-calorie "starvation diets" can cause serious effects in teenagers.

Additionally, low-calorie diets that allow only a few types of foods can be bad for your health because they don't allow you to get enough vitamins and minerals. Kleinman warns that rapid weight loss from very-low-calorie "starvation diets" can cause serious effects in teenagers, such as gallstones, hair loss, weakness, and diarrhea.

Diet Pills

In 1992, FDA banned 111 ingredients in over-the-counter (OTC) diet products—including amino acids, cellulose, and grapefruit extract—after manufacturers were unable to prove that they worked.

A number of products (Cal-Ban 3000, Cal-Lite 1000, Cal-Trim 5000, Perma Slim, Bodi Trim, Dictol 7 Plus, Medi Thin, Nature's Way, and East Indian Guar Gum) were also recalled because they posed serious health risks. The products contained guar gum, which supposedly swelled in the stomach to provide a feeling of fullness. However, the swelling from the guar gum caused blockages in the throat and stomach.

In February 1996, FDA also proposed new warning labels for OTC diet pills containing phenylpropanolamine (PPA), including the statement that the product is "For use by people 18 years of age and older."

PPA is an ingredient found not only in many OTC diet pills but also in cough-cold and allergy products as well. FDA is concerned PPA may possibly increase the risk of a type of stroke (hemorrhagic) caused by bleeding into the brain, as was suggested by some reports of bleeding in the brain among PPA users, typically young women. This possible risk could be further increased if a person took more than the recommended dose of PPA, which might occur inadvertently from also taking a cough-cold product with PPA.

While FDA agrees that studies have not shown a definite link between PPA and stroke, the agency believes data from a more comprehensive study are needed to confirm the ingredient's safety. As a result, the OTC drug industry began a five-year study in 1994.

> A good diet [is] one that has balance, variety and moderation in food choices.

Michael Weintraub, M.D., director of FDA's Office of Drug Evaluation V, says, "PPA is not recommended for use by teenagers also because they are still growing and if they suppress their appetite, they may not get proper nutrition." The author of studies on PPA published in scientific journals, Weintraub adds, "This is especially true of teens who don't need to lose weight but think that they do."

The Real Skinny on Weight Loss

If going to extremes won't do the trick, what will? Believe it or not, it's as simple as making a few changes in your eating habits to emphasize healthy foods and exercise—good advice even if you don't need to lose weight.

Hattner describes a good diet as one that has balance, variety and moderation in food choices. She suggests using the U.S. Department of Agriculture's "Food Pyramid." These guidelines call for six to 11 servings a day of grains (bread, cereal, rice and pasta), three to five servings of vegetables, two to four servings of fruit and two to three servings each of dairy (milk, cheese and yogurt) and protein-rich foods (meat, eggs, poultry, fish, dry beans and nuts).

> Regular exercise . . . is important to look and feel your best.

"The most important dietary change you can make is to limit the amount of high-fat foods that you eat," she adds. "Balance your favorite foods [which are usually high in fat] with fruits and vegetables [which are almost always very low in fat]; eat a wide variety of foods to keep from getting bored and to make sure your diet is nutritionally sound; and keep portion sizes reasonable so that you can have your [thin] slice of cake and lose weight, too."

To keep fat intake down, Hattner recommends making simple lower fat substitutions for the foods that you eat: Switch to 1 percent or skim milk instead of whole milk, nonfat or low-fat frozen yogurt or nonfat or low-fat ice cream instead of regular ice cream, and pretzels instead of corn chips. High-fat foods such as french fries, candy bars, and milkshakes that have no low-fat substitutes should only be eaten once in a while or in very small amounts.

Move It and Lose It

Whether you are overweight or not, regular exercise (at least three times a week) is important to look and feel your best. If you do need to lose weight, stepping up your activity level will cause you to burn calories more quickly and help make weight loss easier.

"Exercise increases lean body weight. Also, you will appear

slimmer as you develop your muscles because muscles give shape and form to your body," notes Hattner.

Fad or starvation diets and diet pills offer temporary solutions, at best. At worst, they may jeopardize your health. According to Weintraub, "The safest way for teenagers to control their weight is to eat a healthy, low-fat diet and get enough exercise."

How Not to Diet

Janis Jibrin

According to Janis Jibrin, a growing number of teenagers are overweight, and many who are not overweight think that they are. She contends that these teenagers often adopt dieting practices that can be dangerous. Jibrin claims that skipping meals, going on low-carbohydrate diets, and taking diet pills are detrimental to a teenager's health. Jibrin is a registered dietician and the author of *The Unofficial Guide to Dieting Safely.*

You may feel desperate to lose weight, but don't fall for these dangerous fads.

A growing number of teens are overweight—11 percent today, compared with 6.5 percent 20 years ago. Still more kids think they're fat, even though they're not. Do you want to drop some pounds? Look out! There are seriously uncool weight-loss approaches out there. Some work for a few weeks, others don't work at all. Even worse, they can crush your self-esteem, stress you out, and harm your health. Here are three weight-loss fads to avoid. Read about them—so you won't fall for them.

Bad Weight Loss Move No. 1: Not Eating All Day

You skip breakfast, then lunch. By afternoon you're starving, but you tell yourself you'll hold off a little longer, then eat a small dinner.

"Kids just can't lose weight this way," says Anne Chasson, a nutritionist from Palo Alto, California. "In fact," says Chasson, "they wind up gaining weight, because as soon as they get home they gorge on everything in sight."

How Fad Diets "Work"

Most of the time, fad diets do not work. Well, sometimes, they may seem to work, at the beginning. Fad diets cannot make up for healthy eating habits.

Some fad diets do not make you lose fat, but make you lose water instead. Many fad diets require pills or food which increase urination. In this way, you will lose water, together with some important vitamins and minerals. . . .

Some other fad diets work, but are unbalanced and lack the taste and nutrition of a healthy diet. You may find it difficult to maintain such an unappealing and boring diet. As time passes, you may lose weight, but soon find yourself gorging on more goodies and gaining more weight than your weight before the fad diet.

Fad diets can be dangerous too and can even lead to death. This is because they lack the nutrients and energy that the body needs. A diet too low in calories may lead to feeling tired, irritable, and experiencing muscle cramps. Lack of protein and carbohydrates can also lead to dizziness, fatigue and other illnesses.

Food Files, "Fad Diets," July 31, 1997.

She's not talking carrot sticks. Those hunger pangs usually send you straight to high-calorie junk like candy, chips, and soda. On this fare it's easy to rack up hundreds, even thousands more calories than if you'd eaten real meals throughout the day.

Eating poorly messes with your head, too. "When kids overeat like this, they wind up depressed, and their self-esteem takes a nose dive," says Chasson. You tell yourself, "Oh, no, I've blown it" and you feel unattractive and unlovable. So, what do you do? Do it all over the next day—both to punish yourself and to blot out the bad feelings.

Bad Weight Loss Move No. 2: High Protein/Low Carb Diet

On this diet, you severely limit high carbohydrate foods like bread, pasta, cereal, potatoes, sweets, and fruit juice. You can eat all the meat, chicken, eggs, cream, and other fats you want. The idea is that without carbohydrates to use as fuel, your body burns stored fat—and you lose weight. Sound like a party?

Well, not really. Weird things start happening to your body when it's deprived of glucose, the fuel it makes from carb-rich foods. Without carbs, your body makes fuel from fat. That fuel is called ketones. Ketones are nasty. They give you bad breath, make you feel dizzy, and some research shows they may cause acid buildup in the bloodstream—which can be lethal.

> [Unhealthy weight loss approaches] can crush your self-esteem, stress you out, and harm your health.

Why do millions of Americans suffer through this ultrapopular diet? Because on the diet, you can lose lots of weight in the first few weeks. But it's water weight, not fat. The weight returns as soon as you start eating carbs again. And you will! Even meat freaks start craving bagels, pasta, and other carbs after being deprived long enough. Then, since you won't have learned how to lose weight on regular food, you'll be back where you started: on your same old fattening diet.

Bad Weight Loss Move No. 3: Pill Popping

There is a pill that makes you burn extra calories and suppresses your appetite. There's just one downside. It can kill you. Ephedrine or Ma Huang (an ephedrine-containing herb) can be found in the diet aisle of most health food stores. Though it may look safe, at least 60 people in the last seven years have died after taking ephedrine. Some of them were teens.

Hundreds of others have suffered heart attacks, strokes, seizures, or attempted suicide after taking the drug. Why? Ephedrine can overstimulate the heart and nervous system, especially in people prone to heart or neurological conditions. Don't take it!

Other diet pills—like Dexatrim and Acutrim—may be just as dangerous. A recent study by a Food and Drug Administration advisory panel found that phenylpropanolamine, an ingredient in every over-the-counter appetite suppressant—increases the risk of stroke in young women by 1,500 percent. The panel recommended that the substance be banned.

Need another reason to skip diet pills? They don't work, unless you eat less or exercise more, and any weight you lose almost always comes back when you stop taking the pills.

Do It Right!

How can you lose weight safely and effectively? Don't diet. Instead, burn calories by becoming more active. It doesn't matter what you do: walking, swimming, biking, dancing, or anything else you like. On the food end, eat more low cal/high nutrient foods like fruits and vegetables, and have smaller portions of high fat/high calorie foods (especially fries, chips, and sodas). And don't even think of dieting if you haven't hit puberty yet (for girls, this means you haven't gotten your period, for boys it means your voice hasn't changed).

Cutting calories may actually stunt your growth! And hang in there. When you hit puberty, weight often drops naturally.

Diet Drug Dangers

Dee Murphy

According to Dee Murphy, many teenagers who want to lose weight take diet pills to suppress their appetites and boost their metabolism. Murphy contends that this practice can be unhealthy because most diet pills, even those prescribed by a doctor, can be harmful to a teenager's health. She maintains that when teenagers suppress their appetites, they reduce their food intake and may not get proper nutrition. Moreover, she alleges that diet pills contain ingredients that affect the cardiovascular and central nervous systems and may cause serious problems such as irregular heart rhythm and increased blood pressure. If you want to lose weight, Murphy suggests that you see a doctor to determine if diet pills are right for you. Murphy is a contributor for *Current Health 2*, a monthly journal that contains information about nutrition, fitness, personal health, drugs, and other health issues for teenagers.

Miracle Diet!
    10 lb Weight Loss this Weekend!
You Will Lose Weight—GUARANTEED!
Diet pills and supplements can promote weight loss, but they

also can carry big health risks. Don't be dazzled by ads promising miracles.

If you've ever wished you could lose a few—or many—pounds in a fast and easy way, chances are you've paid attention to headlines like these in advertisements seen everywhere these days. Even some serious publications run full-page ads that promise, with lots of exclamation marks, that a company's pills, drinks, or supplements will make your extra pounds miraculously melt away.

> Diet pills and supplements . . . can carry big health risks.

Teens seem particularly vulnerable to such ads. They can be influenced by their own self-image—and sometimes subtly by peers, parents, and coaches—to lose weight in order to look good, perform better, or be more popular.

The Centers for Disease Control and Prevention conducted a study of 11,631 high school students and found that more than 43 percent of the girls surveyed said they were "on a diet." The most common dieting methods used were skipping meals, induced vomiting after eating, and taking diet pills. Diet pills can be effective in helping some people lose weight, but are they right for you?

Straight from the Supermarket

Over-the-counter weight-loss drugs such as Acutrim and Dexatrim contain phenyl-propanolamine (PPA), an appetite suppressant that affects the central nervous system. When combined with changes in eating habits and exercise, PPA can help people lose weight. However, the results are temporary and should only be used for the short term (not more than three weeks) until new eating habits are established.

Experts warn that appetite suppressants are most effective in people who are obese, meaning their weight is at least 20 percent over their ideal body weight, as indicated on the body mass index (BMI) [a scale that determines obesity according to a person's height-weight ratio]. Anyone who is only slightly overweight or simply wants to improve his or her appearance should not use these drugs.

In fact, medical experts warn that teens should not take medication containing PPA unless it is ordered and supervised by a doctor. This is the opinion of Michael Weintraub, M.D., who recently served as a director of drug evaluation at the U.S. Food and Drug Administration (FDA). "PPA is not recommended for teens," says Dr. Weintraub, "because they are still growing, and if they suppress their appetites, they may not get proper nutrition." If your doctor does recommend an over-the-counter diet pill, follow his or her dose instructions precisely. PPA can cause severe high blood pressure and an irregular heart rhythm when taken in high doses.

> PPA can cause severe high blood pressure and an irregular heart rhythm.

Are Prescriptions Better?

Even diet pills that are prescribed by a doctor may not be completely safe, either. In 1997, the drugs fenfluramine and dexfenfluramine (the "fen" part of the fen-phen combination often prescribed) were taken off the market. Although these drugs were effective in curbing the appetite, they were linked to heart valve disease as well as a condition called primary pulmonary hypertension. With this condition, there is an increased resistance to blood flow through the lungs. That puts strain on the heart and can lead to heart failure. In October 1999, the company that made Pondimin and Redux (the trade names for the withdrawn drugs) agreed to pay about $4 billion to thousands of people who had evidence that their health was harmed by the drugs.

But new pills have taken their place. Meridia is one such prescription drug that is designed to increase metabolism, cause a feeling of fullness, and increase a person's energy level. Studies show that people who took Meridia had a significant loss of weight, BMI, and waist circumference when they used it along with a low-calorie diet, exercise, and behavior modification. This drug is recommended only for people with a BMI of over 30.

Mike Myers, M.D., a physician in Los Alamitos, California, says that Meridia has its place and can assist with weight loss, but it is not a wonder drug. Meridia's side effects include dry mouth, insomnia, constipation, increase in blood pressure, and a rapid pulse.

What About Herbals?

The latest craze in weight-loss drugs are herbal products that also can carry a risk. Metabolife, Herbal Phen-Fen, and other similar "natural herbals" contain the herbal supplement ephedra, also known as ma huang. Ephedra, chemically related to amphetamine, can have potent side effects. In one case, a 20-year-old Marine became psychotic (afflicted with a serious mental disorder in which one loses contact with reality) while using a supplement containing ephedra. Once he stopped using it, he returned to normal. Other possible side effects include sleeplessness, restlessness, irritability, headache, nausea, vomiting, urinary disorders, and rapid heartbeat. Also, these products can be very dangerous to people with existing health conditions such as high blood pressure.

Overdosing on ephedra can cause a rise in blood pressure, changes in heart rhythm, severe sweating, enlarged pupils, seizures, and fever. Between 1993 and 1997, 34 deaths and 800 medical and psychiatric complications were reported in people using ephedra. Neal Benowitz, M.D., a toxicologist and professor at the University of California at San Francisco, says, "I would prefer to see ephedra pulled off the market until adequate warnings can be developed."

> Ephedra . . . can have potent side effects.

Unlike prescription drugs, herbals are considered dietary supplements, not drugs, and do not go through the FDA approval process for safety and effectiveness. At times, the herbal product doesn't even contain the stated amounts of ingredients on the label. And the manufacturer's claims are usually not confirmed by medical research. "People assume that if it's natural it must be safe," says Gail Mahady, an expert on medicinal plants at the College of Pharmacy at the University of Illinois at Chicago. "But ephedra is a drug."

> Drugs . . . may jeopardize your health.

Metabolism Boosters Can Be Dangerous

Metabolism boosters are often comprised of caffeine and other chemicals (such as ephedrine) that get your heart beating and your energy surging. However, though they may make you lose weight temporarily, there are no studies indicating that they are safe. In fact, many experts agree that metabolism boosters can cause high blood pressure and serious heart problems. Because the more muscle you have, the faster you burn calories, the best way to boost your metabolism is through cardiovascular exercise, which will burn calories and build those muscles at the same time.

Also, contrary to popular belief, eating between meals is also good for your metabolism, because each time you eat, you give your metabolism a little boost. So try to stay away from eating big meals, and eat healthy snacks and smaller portions every couple hours throughout the day.

Kim Rutherford, *TeensHealth*, September 2001.

Herbals and prescription diet pills are designed to be used for the short term to help with lifestyle changes. Drugs alone offer only temporary solutions and, in some cases, may jeopardize your health.

Diet Claims: Fact or Fiction?

When you turn on the television, open the newspaper, or read a magazine, you most likely will find someone promoting a "miracle weight-loss product." These ads claim that the products will help you lose all the weight you want with the least amount of effort. But do they really work, or are these products just full of hot air? Let's look at some manufacturing claims and the truths behind them.

Claim: Lose weight while you sleep.

Fact: Losing weight requires significant changes in the type and amount of food you eat and the burning of calories through increased physical exertion such as exercise. A product that claims weight loss without any kind of sacrifice or effort is bogus.

Claim: Lose weight and keep it off for good.

Fact: Maintaining long-term weight loss requires permanent changes in diet and exercise. Be skeptical about any claim that a product will enable you to keep any weight off permanently.

Claim: John Doe lost 84 pounds in six weeks.

Fact: Just because someone pictured in an ad lost a lot of weight doesn't mean you will, too. Don't be misled.

Claim: Lose all the weight you want for just $99.

> A product that claims weight loss without any kind of sacrifice or effort is bogus.

Fact: You may pay $99 up front, but there are usually hidden costs in the program. For example, some programs don't publicize the fact that you also have to buy prepackaged meals at costs greater than program fees. Before you sign up for any weight-loss program, ask for all the costs in writing.

Claim: Lose 20 pounds in just three weeks.

Fact: As a rule, the faster you lose weight, the faster you gain it back. Plus, fast weight loss can harm your health. Unless you have a medical reason, don't look for programs that promise quick weight loss.

Claim: Scientific breakthrough! Medical miracle!

Fact: Unless the miracle involves reducing your caloric intake and increasing your physical activity, ignore it. The most effective weight-loss programs encourage a modest reduction of food intake of 500 calories per day. At this rate, you will cut 3,500 calories per week, which is equal to one pound of fat. That's a loss that you can live with long-term.

Lies Dieters May Tell Themselves

Kristyn Kusek

In the following article, Kristyn Kusek contends that people trying to lose weight often tell themselves lies that inhibit their weight loss progress. She says that many people believe popular myths such as the idea that combining certain foods burns more calories or that eating low-fat foods will help them lose weight. Kusek maintains that these concepts inhibit weight loss by distracting the dieter from the basic principles of weight loss—if you ingest more calories than you burn, you are going to gain weight. She recommends regular exercise and eating a balanced diet to stay fit. Kusek is a health and lifestyle writer whose work has appeared in *Good Housekeeping* and the *New York Times*.

W ho are you kidding? These white lies may make you feel better now, but they won't help you drop pounds later.

Lie #1: "I Inherited My Weight Problem."

While your parents do have something to do with your weight, you can't blame them for everything. "Your gender, ethnicity, and genes all play a role in your weight," says nutritionist Gail Frank, a spokesperson for the American Dietetic Association. "You may inherit facets of each of your parents' body shapes. If you have your mother's build and she carries extra weight around her stomach, it's likely that you'll get a bit of a tummy if you gain weight too."

But it's the habits your parents passed down that are more likely to affect your weight patterns. "My grandmother and my mother used to walk into the house and eat something while standing over the sink, when they still had their coats on. Those calories didn't count, of course. I do the same thing, and now so do my kids," says Leslie Bonci, director of sports medicine nutrition at the University of Pittsburgh Medical Center. Whether you've inherited weighty genes or pound-adding practices, being overweight doesn't have to be your fate, says Nelda Mercer, a nutritionist in Ann Arbor, MI. "You can make healthy eating choices and become conscious of the bad habits you've learned so that you break the cycle." So just because your mom never exercised doesn't mean you can't make exercise a priority.

Lie #2: "Food Combining Helps Me Burn Calories More Efficiently."

Food combining, a fad that first surfaced in the eighties and lives on in diet books like *The Zone,* has dieters everywhere believing that eating specific ratios of carbohydrates to proteins leads to weight loss. "It's a myth that combining certain foods cranks up your metabolism to burn more calories and pare off pounds," says Frank. Nevertheless, your body does expend more calories digesting certain types of foods. It takes your body the most time and energy to digest fats, such as milk, cheese, and oil. Next come proteins and fiber-rich foods (red meat, eggs, beans). The most rapidly digested foods are simple carbohydrates (sugar, honey, white bread). You'll feel fuller longer if you eat foods that take more time to digest, but because many of these foods are also high in calories, you won't lose weight if you eat more of them. Your best method for burning calories is no surprise: "Eat varied, sensible meals and exercise regularly," says Mercer. "This will give you the most energy, fulfill all of your nutrient requirements (key to keeping your metabolism humming), and help you lose weight in the healthiest way for your body."

Lie #3: "I Don't Have to Exercise to Lose Weight; I Can Just Cut Calories."

You can lose weight without exercising, but you probably won't be able to keep it off. Exercise decreases body fat and increases muscle, and that increases your metabolic rate so you burn more calories even when you're at rest, says Mercer.

Plus, exercise makes you stronger and more fit so you can do activities at a higher intensity and for a longer time, burning even more calories. What all that means: Exercise is just as important to weight loss as cutting calories.

Lie #4: "If I Don't Eat Before I Exercise, I'll Burn More Fat."

Your body needs to have fuel for you to work out at the proper intensity and duration, so it actually is best to eat before you exercise. "If you have lunch at noon, eat nothing for the rest of the day, then exercise after work or school, you probably won't have enough energy to get an efficient, calorie-burning workout," says Bonci. Instead, eat something one to three hours before you exercise, which will give you stamina and prevent you from feeling light-headed and weak during a tough workout. A pre-workout snack can also short-circuit a post-workout binge on fatty foods. (Your metabolism will be slightly elevated after exercise, but not enough to incinerate the bag of chips or candy bar you wolf down because you're famished.) Remember, it's more important to focus on fitting exercise into your daily routine, period, than to worry about how you'll fit it in around your meals.

Lie #5: "If I Eat Only Low-Fat Foods, I'll Lose Weight."

"It's true that cutting fat from your diet can reduce your risk of heart disease, diabetes, and several types of cancer, but it will not ensure weight loss," says Michael Rosenbaum, M.D., an obesity researcher at Columbia Presbyterian Medical Center in New York City. A calorie is a calorie, whether it comes from protein, fat, or carbohydrate. Overloading on fat-free foods can actually backfire on you: Many of them replace the fat with sugar and carbohydrates, increasing the calorie count. These foods also tend to be low in dietary fiber, which has been shown to aid weight control. The American Institute for Cancer Research recommends keeping your fat intake to 15 to 30 percent of total calories, or about 25 to 60 grams a day, depending on how many calories you eat. Even if you're diligent about cutting fat, if you take in more calories than you burn, you're going to gain weight.

Lie #6: "As Long as I Don't Eat After 7 P.M., I'll Lose Weight."

No way. It's not when you eat, but what and how much you eat that's important. (Your body definitely does not store more calories as fat once the sun goes down.) "Ideally you should eat the majority of your calories during the day, when you're the most active, so your body uses the calories for energy instead of storing them as fat; but that doesn't mean you should skip dinner if you get home late from work," says Mercer. Even though you're probably less active in the evening, you're still burning some calories, and it's the total number of calories you consume during a day, week, or month, balanced with the number of calories you burn through activity, that causes weight gain or loss.

Lie #7: "Weighing Myself Every Day Keeps Me on Track."

Once you've begun a weight-loss regimen, don't go near a scale more than once a week. And if you're not trying to lose weight, once a month is sufficient. "There are too many variables, like water retention, that can affect your weight and cause you to be discouraged if you're on a weight-loss program and you weigh yourself daily," says Bonci. "It's healthiest to lose about half a pound a week, so you won't really see any progress if you're stepping on a scale every day." (Most home scales don't detect such small amounts of weight.) Instead, weigh in at the same time, in the same clothes, once a week to get an accurate reading and to stay motivated.

"My Scale Must Be Broken . . ."

No matter what diet fibs you tell yourself, when it comes time to weigh in, the truth comes out—scales don't lie. Here, what really does and doesn't alter that number.

Tall Tale #1: "My Clothes Are Heavy, I'm Deducting Ten Pounds."

THE TRUTH: We'll let you take off two to five pounds. "Depending on the season, shoes generally weigh up to three pounds (one pound for a pair of sandals, three for boots), and the heaviest winter clothes (a sweater and pants) are about two pounds," says nutritionist Leslie Bonci. But to get the most accurate reading when you step on the scale, be consistent: Weigh yourself in the same clothing or while wearing nothing at all.

Tall Tale #2: "I Had a Really Full Bladder, So That Probably Added a Few Pounds."

THE TRUTH: A full bladder adds less than a pound to your weight, and it probably won't even register on your scale. "A cup of water weighs about half a pound, and that much liquid is a pretty full bladder," says nutritionist Gail Frank. "But most home scales weigh pound for pound, so smaller amounts, like a half-pound or a third of a pound, may not show up at all."

Tall Tale #3: "My Hair Was Wet. Subtract Three Pounds."

THE TRUTH: How much wet hair weighs depends on how much hair you have and how wet it is, but it's so unmeasurable that it's not worth worrying about, since wet half is likely to add only a trace amount of weight to any final reading. Once again, consistency counts: If you're used to stepping on the scale right after you get out of the shower, always weigh yourself then.

Tall Tale #4: "I Have Big Breasts—They Must Add Five Pounds to My Weight."

THE TRUTH: "It depends on how blessed you are, but honestly, breasts are not known to be pound powerhouses," says Frank. Breasts may feel heavy, but they probably weigh half a pound to two pounds each, depending on cup size and whether you're pregnant, lactating, or experiencing water retention and swelling because of your period.

Tall Tale #5: "I Can't Weigh That Much! My Scale Is Old (or Broken)."

THE TRUTH: To find out your true weight on your home scale, weigh yourself on a professional scale at your gym or doctor's office, then immediately step on your own scale (in the same clothing) when you get home. That way you can adjust for the difference in what your scale says.

Or invest in a professional scale (one brand: Detecto) that is calibrated to detect smaller segments of weight (like a quarter of a pound). Home scales are just not that sensitive: "If you weigh 130 pounds on your scale, you may actually weigh anywhere from 125 to 135 pounds," says nutritionist Nelda Mercer. "So it's best to pay attention to trends—whether the needle is going up or down—rather than focusing on the number."

A Healthy Weight Loss Plan

Michelle Daum

In the following excerpt from her book *The Can-Do Eating Plan for Overweight Kids and Teens*, pediatric nutritionist Michelle Daum encourages teens to take control of their own eating habits. Teenagers require a lot of calories to grow properly, but Daum contends that some teens eat more calories than their bodies can process. She argues that teens eat outside the home frequently, and they need to learn how to choose healthy, balanced meals. She maintains that by accepting responsibility for their weight loss goals, teenagers can become more healthy and independent.

You're a teenager, which is actually a pretty broad category when it comes to health and fitness. Physically, the body undergoes an extraordinary amount of growth and development during the teen years. In early adolescence, at the onset of puberty, your body requires a great many calories to begin the growth spurt; later, when your physical growth stops and you attain full height, your weight should stabilize. Emotionally, adolescence is a time of increasing independence, and wanting more of a say in what you eat is only natural. So is becoming more concerned about how you look and feel. . . .

Excerpted from *The Can-Do Eating Plan for Overweight Kids and Teens*, by Michelle Daum (New York: Avon Books, 1997). Copyright © 1997 by Michelle Daum. Reprinted by permission of the publisher.

Your Changing Body

I know, I know. It's hard enough to be an adolescent without having to dwell on all the "wonderful" changes your body is going through. But we do have some ground to cover so you can understand the different needs your body has at different stages of adolescence.

Starting at about age ten, your body is gearing up for some extraordinary developments, and caloric needs can be pretty high. This is why parents often joke about how hard it is to keep food in

> You can't expect growth to be a cure-all if you're gaining excessively.

the house with a teenager around. You may in fact feel hungrier than you used to, and that's perfectly normal. When it comes to managing your weight gain as you grow, the trick is to figure out the magic equation that will get you the calories you need to grow while burning excess calories through exercise. While this growth spurt is happening, be careful: It is still possible to out-gain your growth. You can't expect growth to be a cure-all if you're gaining excessively. You will not outgrow the overweight with which you entered adolescence—at least not without making some significant lifestyle changes.

For girls, the onset of menstrual periods (around age twelve and a half) marks the end of rapid growth. A girl may continue to slowly grow another inch or two over the next year or two, but seldom more than that. So her caloric intake will need to slow down at that time or she will start to gain weight excessively. She can no longer count on growth to counteract overeating.

After your growth spurt has stopped, you have attained your full height, and your weight gain should stabilize. Because you won't be getting any taller, you don't need to keep eating as much to keep up with increasing inches. Instead, with your doctor's help, you want to determine your ideal weight and eat just enough to fuel your body's daily activities without overeating.

The Teen Lifestyle

As a teen, you are more likely to be eating outside your home. Schedules get complicated, and eating out may be the main kind of eating you do. You might pick up breakfast on the way to school, grab a snack from the vending machine between classes, head out for fast food with friends at lunch, and indulge in a slice or two of pizza in the afternoon before dinner. Those extra calories can really add up, especially once you've stopped growing taller. At the end of each day, you have more homework than you used to, and you may develop the habit of snacking while studying, which means still more calories.

If you have a job, you may be around food all the time, in a restaurant, a snack bar, or ice cream parlor. Baby-sitting is another opportunity for overindulging; after putting the kids to bed, there's a real temptation to snack until the parents return (I remember doing this in my baby-sitting days!). Whatever your job, with that extra spending money burning a hole in your pocket, you'll be able to buy snacks whenever you choose.

You are probably socializing more independently, too. And, let's face it, eating is a big part of the social scene for all of us. You go to the mall and have lunch. You get popcorn and soft drinks at the movies. You have a cookout at the end of softball season. You go on a dinner date. It's just a way of life. Dances, parties, bar and bat mitzvahs, sweet-sixteen celebrations—all of these can center around food, and that's hard when you're watching your weight. Even when there's dancing or some other activity, it's hard to avoid the snack table.

> Eating is almost incidental to hanging out.

Eating is almost incidental to hanging out. You don't want to stick close to home, so you get together with your group of friends and order Cokes and fries or nachos or ice cream, and it can go on for hours. Even if you've been aware of your weight problem for a while, you may have found it hard to "just say no" when you're out with the gang. . . . [Here are some suggestions to help you avoid overeating in social situations.]

• Have a small meal before a party so you're not as eager to dive into the snack trays.

• Limit yourself to one soft drink or other beverage. After that, stick to water.

• If you're asked to bring a snack, select a lower-calorie option . . . such as popcorn, pretzels, or even a watermelon.

> You didn't put the weight on overnight, and you can't lose it overnight.

• At a cookout, team banquet, or other buffet, have first helpings only—no seconds or thirds.

• Bring your own snacks to the movies—and don't be lured by popcorn, which is very high in calories. You could buy a movie snack and eat only part of it, or agree to share with a friend.

About Alcohol

Teenagers are forbidden by law from drinking alcoholic beverages. But despite the risks—not the least of which is a drunk-driving accident—many still do. I strongly urge any underage person to avoid drinking alcohol. If you are overweight, you have still another reason to abstain: Alcoholic beverages of all kinds—beer, wine, and liquor—are extremely high in calories and are not in any way a part of [a healthy weight-loss] plan.

Your Personal Weight Goals

Social pressures increase during the teenage years. You're attending a larger school, your classmates are starting to separate into different groups or cliques, and you wonder where you fit in. If you suspect you have a weight problem, you may feel quite sensitive. You're not alone.

Many teenagers who come to me have a very specific goal:

I want to lose two dress sizes by the prom in June.

I need to be down fifteen pounds by basketball tryouts.

I should reduce my waist three inches before I leave for college.

I have to drop ten pounds before swim team practice starts.

Sound familiar? The truth is, adults are pretty much the same way. And I tell them exactly the same thing: You didn't put the weight on overnight, and you can't lose it overnight, no matter what they tell you on television. Still, everybody seems to think there's some instant solution.

There *is* a solution, but it isn't instant, so you'll need to make a strong commitment to this new way of life. It won't be as hard as it sounds, because the foods in [a healthy weight-loss] plan are pretty much the same foods you already enjoy. But you'll eat less of them. And you'll need to burn more calories with regular exercise.

About Exercise

Team sports are popular with adolescents, and they offer the advantage of regular scheduling: You go to school, you go to sports, and then you go home, without having to make extra time for exercise. If you are into sports, make sure to keep working out in some way even between seasons (walk, jog, or use a workout tape or some sports equipment). The three weeks between football and basketball seasons is plenty of time to lose ground where conditioning is concerned.

If team sports aren't your thing, you're not alone. There are many options for the nonathlete. Physical fitness doesn't mean becoming an expert tennis player. It means improving your strength, endurance, and flexibility. How? By getting at least thirty minutes of good, heart-pumping aerobic exercise three times a week or more. That is what will burn those extra calories. Exercise is also a proven stress buster—and with the pressures of adolescence, it's a safe bet you could use some relief! (In fact, some of you may be consuming extra calories in response to stress, which certainly increases as you reach your teen years.)

Unfortunately, exercise alone is not always enough. You may be on the baseball team, but if you're an outfielder, you're not moving around very much. Soccer can be great exercise, but if you're the goalie, you may or may not be working hard. In these situations, you can supplement with additional exercise. Whatever activity you choose should keep you breathing rapidly and moving your muscles for thirty minutes or more. Work up a sweat!

If you need a motivator, try enlisting a friend to become your workout buddy. You'll be less likely to cancel plans for a walk or an aerobics class when you know someone's counting on you. And it's always more fun to have a friend along.

Travel Temptations

You're on your own, traveling with a group, participating in an exchange program or summer enrichment program, working as a camp counselor or mother's helper, and your food choices change. Eating opportunities may be limited: Your host family feeds you or you eat meals in a cafeteria or your tour group stops at a fast-food restaurant. Perhaps your opportunities to eat may be unlimited: You're on your own, choosing when and what to eat. Either way, your options are

> Exercise is . . . a proven stress buster.

harder to control than when you're at home. Learning to make choices that fit your weight-management goals will keep you on track. Take smaller portions, eat less of the portion you're served, work in extra exercise, fill up on lower-calorie items. (This is an excellent way to deal with restaurant meals in general. Remember, just because they've served it to you doesn't mean you have to clean your plate!)

Off to College

You may have heard about the Freshman Fifteen—the legendary "automatic weight gain" that all new college students are said to endure. How does it happen? Think about it. You're completely on your own for the first time, eating with friends in the cafeteria for breakfast, lunch, and dinner, often prolonging the meal by socializing. You're snacking in your room; because most dorms don't allow cooking, snack foods are easiest to store. Supermarkets may be inaccessible to you, forcing you to buy junk food at the campus convenience store. And everytime you turn around, someone's ordering pizza. By winter break, you've gained weight.

> Just because they've served it to you doesn't mean you have to clean your plate!

The good news is that your college roommates and other friends are going through it, too. And together, you can come up with some solutions. Organize an aerobics group or take an exercise class together. Play an intramural sport. Walk to class instead of taking the campus bus (or get off the bus a few stops early and walk the rest of the way). Or ride a bike! Make frequent use of the athletic center. Agree to help each other to limit high-calorie snacking to one or two nights a week or fewer. . . . And whatever you do, don't starve yourself to stay thinner by going on a crash diet. Even if your body is full grown, it still needs calories to perform efficiently. See your doctor to determine the appropriate weight goal for you, from among three options: weight slowdown, weight maintenance, and weight loss (only for full-grown teens or severely obese growing kids). Only your doctor will be able to tell you how much more growing you are likely to do, and what you should do about your weight now. . . .

It's All in the Timing

If you're like most teens, you are active day to night, all week long, waking up early for school, going nonstop with classes, homework, activities, and socializing. On weekends, you may "crash," sleeping in and disrupting your eating schedule. Because you're so busy, you have many opportunities to snack throughout the day, opportunities you may not even think about, like eating chips as you study, grabbing an ice cream with a friend, drinking a soda at a sports event. And because you're becoming independent, making your own plans and spending your own money, it will be up to you to set limits. [You need to create] a framework for eating that includes three meals a day plus snacks. You can then decide for yourself if you want a dessert right after dinner or something to munch on later as you finish homework or watch a video. And when unexpected snacking opportunities arise—a class party, pizza with friends—you can remind yourself to give up one of your scheduled snacks in exchange. (Getting extra exercise that day also helps!) You really don't need to say no to the normal socializing that all teenagers enjoy. All it takes is some moderation, some give and take. In time, you'll find it becoming easier to set limits for yourself.

> Don't starve yourself to stay thinner by going on a crash diet.

At Mom's House, at Dad's House

Taking control of your eating in your every day environment is one thing, but what about the time you spend outside your usual routine? If your parents are divorced, you may confront some challenges when you spend a night, a weekend, or a vacation with the parent you see less often. Going out to eat may be a regular part of your visit, and it will be up to you to set some limits on what you order and how much you eat. If that parent lives far enough away from your other parent that you can't see your friends or visit your regular hang-outs, it may be easy to slip away from your everyday regimen. If you can, why not enlist the help of both parents? Talk about your new way of eating. Find out about exercise opportunities near each parent's home (local recreation classes, aerobics studios, even hiking trails). You can even make plans for some physical activity you can do together with each of them.

Increasing independence is one of the perks of growing up. It is, as they say, a privilege and a responsibility. You have the privilege of making more of your own decisions. And you have a responsibility to make the best decisions you can. For this reason, I encourage adolescents to be in charge of their own weight management. You're not a kid anymore, and you don't need your mom and dad to play "food police" while you get annoyed and try to undermine them. It's too easy for you to get those extra calories when you're out and about. And it's wrong for your parents to battle with you over what you ate when, and how much. Make this *your* project. After all, you are the one who will benefit.

It's certainly fine to ask for support from your parents as you embark on this lifestyle change, however. Here are some ways your parents can help you:

• Have your parents make an appointment with your doctor, who can perform a physical examination to see where things stand right now and help you select a weight-management goal and a calorie level. . . .

• Make a list of the items you want to keep around the house for your breakfasts, lunches, and snacks. (If you drive, perhaps your parent would allow you to go out and purchase the items yourself.)

• Talk about ways to get exercise, such as taking a class, working out with an exercise video, riding a bicycle, and so on. Discuss which options appeal to you, and how often they will be available. You will want to exercise three or more times a week for at least thirty minutes per session, so be sure to choose something you'll be able to do regularly.

Your parents want to be an emotional support for you. But don't ask them to be your keepers. If you aren't ready to make a change, there's nothing your parents can do to make you watch your weight. Temptations are everywhere. That's why you'll have to take charge. This is your chance to be independent. . . . Don't rely on your parents to tell you no. Those days are over. Now it's up to you.

Point of Contention: Can Fad Diets Promote Weight Loss?

Dieticians and nutritionists maintain that nearly 90 percent of people who lose weight gain it back within five years. Health experts contend that the best way to lose weight and keep it off is to slowly decrease caloric intake and increase physical activity. However, this process of weight loss requires substantial changes in lifestyle and promises weight loss of only one to two pounds per week. Many dieters get frustrated with the day-to-day monitoring of calories and fat intake and seek quick remedies. This frustration has spawned a multibillion-dollar dieting industry that offers books, pills, foods, programs, and miracles that promise quick weight loss with minimal effort. The most recent dieting fads include high-protein, low-carbohydrate diets, herbal weight loss pills, and food-combining (a theory that food eaten in certain combinations can speed weight loss).

Health professionals argue that fad diets and quick-fix remedies do not work because although dieters may lose weight quickly, they will regain the weight once they start eating normally. Moreover, these experts allege that fad diets lack essential nutrients and can cause health problems. Diet gurus disagree and maintain that their programs are healthy, safe, and effective at promoting weight loss. The following articles reflect this debate over weight loss. Nutrition and health writer Catherine Houck argues that a short-term crash diet can facilitate weight loss. In contrast, nutritional counselor and medical writer Cindy Maynard contends that fad diets pose serious health risks.

Fad Diets Can Promote Weight Loss

Catherine Houck

We all know dieting is passe. Instead of fretting over those calorie counts, you're supposed to be making healthy lifestyle changes. But you also know that the scale has been firmly stuck at that not-so-great number [for a long time].

What your body just might need is a jump-start, the kind of quick drop in weight that gives you a powerful mental boost. Maybe most of those pounds lost will be water weight, and maybe the scale will creep back up a little, post-victory. Yo-yo weight fluctuation is what gives fads like the Cabbage Soup Diet a bad name.

Nonetheless, sometimes we need to see some real progress at the start of a diet to motivate us through the day-in, day-out sensible regimen of keeping portions down; curbing intake of fatty, sugary, and salty foods; and staying active. "Research suggests that from a psychological perspective, fast weight loss early on can predict longer-term success," says Karen Miller-Kovach, R.D., lead scientist for Weight Watchers International.

Is it possible to shed pounds swiftly yet safely? If your crash diet doesn't last longer than seven days, nutritional needs won't have to be sacrificed, say diet experts. "You do have to accept that it won't be a pleasure diet," says Yolanda Bergman, a Hollywood diet guru. "But you won't be faint with hunger—and a week isn't that long."

Depending on your weight when you start out, you can

expect to lose up to five pounds by following this plan. The further you are from your ideal weight, the more you'll lose. If your diet's been very salty, you'll drop faster too. "Some of the loss will be water, but that's fine, because water bloat comes out of your face," says Stephen Gullo, Ph.D., a psychologist and weight-control expert. "That way, you'll start looking visibly thinner in three or four days." And chances are, you'll feel a lot lighter.

> Sometimes we need to see some real progress at the start of a diet to motivate us.

Avoid the Starving-Yourself Trap

Don't go more than four hours without eating a meal or a snack—fasting leads to bingeing all too often. "The best way to prevent cravings is to make sure you don't go hungry," says Gullo. Recommended snacks include nonfat fruit-flavored yogurt and a piece of whole wheat toast with a small amount of fat-free cream cheese. At dinner, try a smart first course to keep the main meal small. A study from the department of psychiatry and behavioral sciences at Johns Hopkins University School of Medicine found that a bowl of tomato soup "significantly" reduced the size of the next course.

Menus should be planned ahead. Knowing what's to be eaten prevents having to make food decisions when you're vulnerable. "Plan what not to eat too," says Gullo. "Clear your house of foods you have a history of abusing—cookies, chips, chocolate, peanuts, ice cream, whatever is your trigger."

Hit the Green-and-White Basics

"Green" means vegetables—lettuce, spinach, kale, peas, broccoli, green beans, asparagus, watercress, zucchini, and cabbage. "White" means certain lean proteins—turkey, chicken, shrimp, crab, scallops, fish fillets, egg whites, tuna, tofu. "You can't go wrong eating mostly vegetables and low-fat protein," says Gullo. "It's an eating plan high in nutrients and low in calories, and the vegetable fiber takes the place of fat as an appetite suppressor."

Try to consume at least five servings of vegetables a day, striving for as many different kinds as possible. A March 1999 study conducted by the Energy Metabolism Laboratory at Tufts University found that the subjects who ate the widest variety of vegetables had the least amount of body fat. For protein, eat at least two servings a day—a serving means four to six ounces of seafood, four ounces of chicken or turkey, or eight ounces of yogurt.

A good way to combine vegetables and protein is stir-frying; to cut down on preparation time, use precut chicken and shelled, deveined shrimp, along with prechopped frozen or fresh onions, bell peppers, other veggies, and garlic. To cook, you need only a thin layer of cooking spray in a nonstick pan; add just a touch of an assertive oil such as hot chili or toasted sesame, and herbs and spices such as cumin, oregano, or thyme. If food sticks, splash in a few tablespoons of broth or wine.

> Don't go more than four hours without eating a meal or a snack.

Curb the Carbs

As anyone who has read Dr. Robert C. Atkins's *New Diet Revolution* knows, a vital part of many of the latest diets is restricting starchy carbohydrates. For this plan, just one a day is recommended. "Eating a lot of crackers, bagels, pasta, sugary cereals and desserts, white rice, and white bread adds little to nutrition but does a lot to prevent weight loss," says Bergman. "Make even your once-a-day serving as natural and unprocessed as possible—brown rice, oatmeal, whole grains." Potatoes are also a good choice. A study from the department of biochemistry at the University of Sydney in Australia found that out of 38 foods, boiled potatoes made people feel the most full (croissants ranked the lowest on the same scale).

Make sure to have two pieces of fruit a day, but no more, during your one-week crash. Fruit is important for its fiber and phyto-chemicals, but Gullo is one expert who believes more than two servings slows weight loss. Avoid finger fruits such as grapes, or bowls of cut-up fruit. Although they're fine nutritionally, it's too easy to lose track of how much you're eating. "Stick with whole fruit—apples, oranges, pears, peaches, nectarines," Gullo advises.

> You can't go wrong eating mostly vegetables and low-fat protein.

Watch the Bloat Factor

The best strategy is to gently adjust the body's fluid by eating less salt, says Miller-Kovach. (Over-the-counter diuretics can cause dehydration, muscle cramps, even cardiac arrhythmia.) But just removing the salt shaker isn't enough—85 percent of the salt we eat is contained in processed foods. Everybody knows cold cuts and pickles are loaded, but so is bread. Ditto breakfast cereals, cheese (including cottage cheese), frozen dinners, crackers, and vegetable juices (unless they're the "low sodium" kind). On fixed labels, anything with the word sodium has salt. "The best way to cut salt is to eat produce, proteins, and grains in their most simple, natural state, without sauces and dressings," says Miller-Kovach.

Ratchet Up the Workout

The prevailing wisdom is that if you increase your activity but don't watch your calories, you probably won't lose weight. If you restrict calories but don't exercise, you'll likely drop some pounds, but not enough to run out and buy those slinky black pants. To shed the most weight in the least time, you must increase exercise and decrease calories.

"If you're walking three times a week for twenty minutes, make it six times for forty minutes," says Bergman. Gabe Mirkin, M.D., associate professor of sports medicine at Georgetown Medical School, goes even further. "The longer you work out, the more calories you burn," he says. Runners who finish last in marathons use more calories than runners who cross the finish line first. The same thing applies to all forms of exercise: To lose weight fast, get out and walk vigorously for 60 minutes if you are accustomed to moderate workouts. If not, break the walks into four 15-minute segments to prevent injuries.

Another way to speed up calorie loss, sometimes dramatically, is to switch to a different kind of workout. If you've been a walker, take up bicycling; if you've been bicycling, change to aerobic dance. Muscles get extremely efficient at constantly performing the same jobs, and this efficiency decreases the calories needed to do the activities, explains Robert McMurray, Ph.D., professor of exercise and sports science at the University of North Carolina, Chapel Hill. Switching to a workout that uses different muscles increases calorie burn.

85 percent of the salt we eat is in processed foods.

However much exercise you're able to do, there's some evidence that extra calories can be burned by doing it early in the day and outdoors. Exercising in natural morning light speeds up metabolism, which otherwise rises slowly throughout the morning, says Timothy Monk, Ph.D., director of the Human Chronobiology Research Program at the University of Pittsburgh School of Medicine. "Even a ten-minute walk to work helps."

A New Way of Eating

It's easy to be so delighted by the rapid loss of a few pounds that you decide to keep on going. "This is usually a bad idea," says Miller-Kovach. "It's not difficult to live austerely for a week, but having no end in sight changes the psychological landscape. You put yourself at high risk of a deprivation/binge cycle that will bring back all the lost weight."

After the week is up, stay active and continue a diet that features lots of vegetables and low-fat protein, but increase the amount of carbs to lose at a "keep it off" rate of one pound a week. Feel free to eat more fruit. Miller-Kovach says, "Fruits are so low in calories, I've yet to meet anyone capable of fruit abuse." Overall, most women should consume at least 1,200 calories per day. "Mainly, be persistent," says Gullo. "If you slip, return to healthy, moderate eating the next day. Don't let a single mistake with a glob of calories undermine what you've accomplished."

From "The Crash Diet That Works—Honest!" by Catherine Houck, *Good Housekeeping*, November 1999. Copyright © 1999 by Catherine Houck. Reprinted with permission.

Fad Diets Can Be Unhealthy

Cindy Maynard

If you're trying to lose weight, here's what you should know about the popular diets at the moment.

"Lose 30 pounds in 30 days." "Medical Miracle!" "Burn, block, flush fat from your system!"

These ads shout at you from TV and radio commercials, magazines, and newspapers. Walk into any bookstore and you'll probably see a new diet book on the shelves. There's *Enter the Zone, Sugar Busters, Dr. Atkins' New Diet Revolution,* and books about liquid diets. A few years ago carbohydrates were the dieter's best friend. Now protein reigns as the new star.

> 15 to 35 percent of Americans are trying to lose weight.

Each new remedy is greeted with a wave of enthusiasm. And yet, these "miracle diets" come and go like miniskirts, platform shoes, and celebrity romances. They're condemned by health professionals because they're dangerous, or people can't stay on them because they're so boring. Another one comes along and we say, "Maybe this one will work." After all, they claim to be the newest, the best, the most effective. Right? But which ones are healthy and which ones are hype?

A Nation of Dieters

Americans, including teens, are desperate to lose weight. As you read this, an amazing 15 to 35 percent of Americans are trying to lose weight. Obesity is a reality in our country. The health risks associated with overweight and obesity—such as high blood pressure, diabetes, stroke, and some cancers—are well-known. Here are some other facts to chew on:

• Ninety-five percent of all dieters will regain their lost weight in one to five years.

• Eighty-one percent of 10-year-olds are afraid of being fat.

• Thirty-five percent of "normal dieters" progress to pathological dieting or full-blown eating disorders.

• Americans spend more than $40 billion on dieting and diet-related products each year.

In spite of these statistics, America is becoming fatter. Obesity has risen to 33 percent of the population, up from 25 percent in the 1980s. This makes the lure of quick, easy weight-loss schemes hard to resist. But there

> Dieting lowers lean muscle mass, which lowers metabolism.

are some good reasons why fad diets aren't healthy and don't work for the long haul. Let's look at some of the most popular diets.

The Latest Skinny on Dieting

Dieting lowers lean muscle mass, which lowers metabolism. The brain recognizes the starvation mode and tells the body to start "storing fat." This is why it becomes harder to lose weight.

• Fad diets typically lack energy (calories) and one or more nutrients essential for health.

• Fad diets can keep a teen from growing properly. They can make girls, especially athletes with low body fat, stop menstruating and boys stop developing muscles.

• Fad diets are boring. Is this spartan regime really something you can maintain the rest of your life? Let's get real.

Before you jump on the diet bandwagon, consider these facts about the latest weight-loss crazes.

High-Protein/Low-Carb Diets

The assumption here is that many people suffer a carbohydrate allergy. When they eat sugar or carbohydrates, the thinking goes, their bodies produce more insulin, which increases fat storage and appetite. A person on a high-protein diet is allowed to eat high saturated fat and cholesterol-laden foods like meat, eggs, and butter, but he or she must avoid fresh fruits, grains, and starchy vegetables. This diet may work in the short run as long as the person is cutting back on calories and exercising. But its high-protein content has no effect on the weight loss. The high-protein diet is not healthy in the long run, though. It lacks fiber, phyto-chemicals, vitamins, and minerals known to help prevent cancer, heart disease, and osteoporosis. Lack of fiber can cause problems such as constipation, dehydration, weakness, and nausea. It can also put a strain on the kidneys.

Liquid Diets

These over-the-counter or medically supervised liquid meal diet plans should not be used for long-term weight loss. This is a regime that's used as a last resort for chronically obese persons, and it may lack essential nutrients for growth, which could compromise your health. It does not teach new eating habits and behavior, which are necessary for maintaining weight loss.

Fasting and Very Low-Calorie Diets

Many people use fasting to cleanse the body of toxins or to start a new weight-loss program. Fasting for weight loss starves the body of energy and nutrients. Very low-calorie diets compromise health and slow down your metabolism. You may lose weight initially, but it's mostly water and lean muscle tissue, not fat. Like the other diets, fasting does not teach new or permanent healthier eating habits.

Healthy Tips to Help Lose Weight

If fad diets don't work, what does? Here are some tips that most experts can agree upon:

• Focus on a lower-fat diet with the emphasis on whole grains and more fresh fruits and vegetables daily.

• Move your body. The latest research shows any kind of physical movement is better than none, even if it is for just 10 minutes a day.

• Make dietary and fitness changes slowly so the habit "sticks." Choose one goal, such as replacing one soda a day with low-fat milk or adding one more serving of vegetables. Even small changes can make a difference.

• Practice guilt-free eating, and savor the textures and flavors of the foods you consume. Eating should always be a pleasure.

Fad Diets Cut Out Nutrients

If people can't stay on a fad diet, and if they regain the weight they've lost once they end it, they might as well not have tried it in the first place. Then there's the health aspect. In addition to carbohydrates, many of today's popular diets say no to fruits and vegetables. That's strange, given that (1) an estimated one-third of all cancers are related to diet, and (2) the good guys in the cancer-fighting equation are the very foods the fad diets rule out. Fruits and vegetables contain vitamin C, folic acid, fiber, and many other nutrients that researchers believe protect against cancer. It's also pretty well agreed that other plant chemicals known as phytochemicals—lycopene in tomatoes, isothiocyanates in broccoli, genestein in soybeans, and allyl sulfides in garlic and onions, to name a few—also play a protective role. Supplements are fine, but we'll never be able to pack all those nutrients into a pill.

Donald Hensrud, *Fortune,* May 15, 2000.

• Keep a food journal of what you're eating. It's easier to examine your eating habits once you write them down.

• Get a coach. It's not always easy to determine what foods to eat to achieve your goals. If you require more support, go to a registered dietitian.

Kathryn Schulz, 17, of Woodbridge High School in Irvine, California, says, "Most people know fad diets don't work, but everyone wants an easy solution, so they pop this wonder pill because it sounds good. Fad diets cause you to binge eat. Talk to a doctor or dietitian instead of listening to a fashion magazine. Try to eat healthy and exercise. You'll get a lot better results than from a shake or pill."

Diet or Disorder? It's a Thin Line

What about the teen who takes dieting to the extreme? Many teens who are at a healthy weight believe they are obese, so they adopt bizarre diet patterns that can trigger disordered eating. The consequences can be devastating.

That's not news to Tara Sharpell, 15, from Escondido, California. She is a client of Healthy Within, an intensive day treatment program for women with anorexia and bulimia in San Diego, California. "After a while you lose out because you can lose weight and go too far and get an eating disorder," she says. "I lost so much more than the weight. I paid a high price. Focus on what you really want. Is this diet really going to give you a perfect body? Will the diet fix all the problems? Probably not."

The high-protein diet is not healthy in the long run.

Dr. Divya Kakaiya, Ph.D., director of Healthy Within, agrees. "For many teenagers, dieting can be a very normal activity of adolescence," she says. "Eating disorders commonly start with a dieting attempt at some point in high school. The biggest message I'd like to give young girls [and guys] is to resist the peer pressure of dieting."

Do you have a friend or family member who seems to be struggling with an eating disorder? If so, encourage him or her to seek professional help.

What's a Body to Do?

Everyone deserves to feel good about themselves now, rather than waiting for some elusive day the scale hits the right weight. Focus on what you want. Is it athletics, top-notch performance, a positive body image, feeling creative or energetic? Fad diets are not the way to go for any of these goals.

Remember: We're given only one body. We can't exchange it for a new one. So be good to it.

From "Fad Diets: A Reality Check," by Cindy Maynard, *Current Health 2*, January 2000. Copyright © 2000 by Weekly Reader Corporation. Reprinted with permission.

Organizations and Websites

The editors have compiled the following list of organizations concerned with the issues debated in this book. The descriptions are derived from materials provided by the organizations. All have publications or information available for interested readers. The list was compiled on the date of publication of the present volume; the information provided here may change. Be aware that many organizations take several weeks or longer to respond to inquiries, so allow as much time as possible.

American Academy of Child and Adolescent Psychiatry (AACAP)

3615 Wisconsin Ave. NW, Washington, DC 20016
(202) 966-7300 • fax: (202) 966-2891
website: www.aacap.org

AACAP is a nonprofit organization dedicated to providing parents and families with information regarding developmental, behavioral, and mental disorders that affect children and adolescents. The organization provides national public information through the distribution of the newsletter *Facts for Families* and the monthly *Journal of the American Academy of Child and Adolescent Psychiatry*.

American Anorexia/Bulimia Association, Inc. (AA/BA)

165 W. 46th St., Suite 1108, New York, NY 10036
(212) 575-6200
e-mail: amanbu@aol.com
website: http://members.aol.com/amanbu

AA/BA is a nonprofit organization that works to prevent eating disorders by informing the public about their prevalence, early warning signs, and symptoms. AA/BA also provides information about effective treatments to sufferers and their families and friends.

American Psychiatric Association (APA)
1400 K St. NW, Washington, DC 20005
(202) 682-6000 • fax: (202) 682-6850
e-mail: apa@psych.org • website: www.psych.org

APA is an organization of psychiatrists dedicated to studying the nature, treatment, and prevention of mental disorders. It helps create mental health policies, distributes information about psychiatry, and promotes psychiatric research and education. APA publishes the monthly *American Journal of Psychiatry.*

American Psychological Association
750 First St. NE, Washington, DC 20002-4242
(202) 336-5500 • fax: (202) 336-5708
e-mail: public.affairs@apa.org • website: www.apa.org

This society of psychologists aims to "advance psychology as a science, as a profession, and as a means of promoting human welfare." It produces numerous publications, including the monthly journal *American Psychologist,* the monthly newspaper *APA Monitor,* and the quarterly *Journal of Abnormal Psychology.*

Anorexia Nervosa and Bulimia Association (ANAB)
767 Bayridge Dr., PO Box 20058, Kingston, ON K7P 1CO
Canada
website: www.phe.queensu.ca/anab

ANAB is a nonprofit organization made up of health professionals, volunteers, and past and present victims of eating disorders and their families and friends. The organization advocates and coordinates support for individuals affected directly or indirectly by eating disorders. As part of its effort to offer a broad range of current information, opinion, and/or advice concerning eating disorders, body image, and related issues, ANAB produces the quarterly newsletter *Reflections.*

Anorexia Nervosa and Related Eating Disorders, Inc. (ANRED)

PO Box 5102, Eugene, OR 97405

(503) 344-1144

website: www.anred.com

ANRED is a nonprofit organization that provides information about anorexia nervosa, bulimia nervosa, binge eating disorder, compulsive exercising, and other lesser-known food and weight disorders, including details about recovery and prevention. ANRED offers workshops, and individual and professional training, as well as local community education. It also produces a monthly newsletter.

Eating Disorders Awareness and Prevention, Inc. (EDAP)

603 Stewart St., Suite 803, Seattle, WA 98101

(206) 382-3587 • fax: (206) 292-9890

website: www.nationaleatingdisorders.org

EDAP is dedicated to promoting the awareness and prevention of eating disorders by encouraging positive self-esteem and size acceptance. It provides free and low-cost educational information on eating disorders and their prevention. EDAP also provides educational outreach programs and training for schools and universities and sponsors the Puppet Project for Schools and the annual National Eating Disorders Awareness Week. EDAP publishes a prevention curriculum for grades four through six as well as public prevention and awareness information packets, videos, guides, and other materials.

Harvard Eating Disorders Center (HEDC)
356 Boylston St., Boston, MA 02118
(888) 236-1188

HEDC is a national nonprofit organization dedicated to research and education. It works to expand knowledge about eating disorders and their detection, treatment, and prevention and promotes the healthy development of women, children, and everyone at risk. A primary goal for the organization is lobbying for health policy initiatives on behalf of individuals with eating disorders.

National Association of Anorexia and Associated Disorders (ANAD)
Box 7, Highland Park, IL 60035
hot line: (847) 831-3438 • fax: (847) 433-4632
e-mail: anad20@aol.com
website: www.anad.org

ANAD offers hot-line counseling, operates an international network of support groups for people with eating disorders and their families, and provides referrals to health-care professionals who treat eating disorders. It produces a quarterly newsletter and information packets and organizes national conferences and local programs. All ANAD services are provided free of charge.

National Eating Disorder Information Centre (NEDIC)
CW 1–211, 200 Elizabeth St., Toronto, ON M5G 2C4 Canada
(416) 340-4156 • fax: (416) 340-4736
e-mail: mbeck@torhosp.toronto.on.ca • website: www.nedic.on.ca

NEDIC provides information and resources on eating disorders and weight preoccupation, and it focuses on the sociocultural factors that influence female health-related behaviors. NEDIC promotes healthy lifestyles and encourages individuals to make informed choices based on accurate information. It publishes a newsletter and a guide for families and friends of eating-disorder sufferers and sponsors Eating Disorders Awareness Week in Canada.

National Eating Disorders Organization (NEDO)

6655 S. Yale Ave., Tulsa, OK 74136

(918) 481-4044

website: www.kidsource.com/nedo

NEDO provides information, prevention, and treatment resources for all forms of eating disorders. It believes that eating disorders are multidimensional, developed and sustained by biological, social, psychological, and familial factors. It publishes information packets, a video, and a newsletter, and it holds a semiannual national conference.

Society for Adolescent Medicine (SAM)

1916 NW Copper Oaks Circle, Blue Springs, MO 64015

(816) 224-8010

website: www.adolescenthealth.org

SAM is a multidisciplinary organization of professionals committed to improving the physical and psychosocial health and well-being of all adolescents. It helps plan and coordinated national and international professional education programs on adolescent health. Its publications include the monthly *Journal of Adolescent Health* and the quarterly *SAM Newsletter*.

Websites

Dear Lucie

www.lucie.com

Lucie Walters writes a syndicated newspaper and online advice column for teens called *Adolessons*. Her columns discuss eating disorders, dieting, health, body image, and other teen issues. Visitors to the site can read archives of her columns as well as participate in message boards and chat rooms.

Teen Advice Online (TAO)

www.teenadviceonline.org

TAO's teen counselors from around the world offer advice for teens on health, fitness, dieting, body image, family, school, substance abuse, dating, sex and sexuality, gender issues, and relationships. Teens can submit questions to the counselors or read about similar problems in the archives.

Teen Advice.Net

teenadvice.studentcenter.org

Teen Advice.Net offers students and teens expert and peer advice about health, body image, relationships, sexuality, gender issues, and other teen concerns. The webpage was created by the Student Center, a web community for college students, high school students, and teenagers.

Whole Family

www.wholefamily.com

This source is designed for both parents and teens. The site's advice columnist, Liz, answers questions about body image, dieting, fitness, teen sex, drugs, drinking, and pregnancy, while online articles discuss other issues such as divorce, relationships, and health.

Bibliography

Books

Arnold Anderson
Making Weight: Healing Men's Conflicts with Food, Weight, and Shape. San Diego: Gurze, 2000.

Katie S. Bagley
Eat Right: Tips for Good Nutrition. Mankato, MN: Capstone, 2001.

Karen Belliner
Diet Information for Teens. Holmes, PA: Omnigraphics, 2001.

Frances Berg
Afraid to Eat. Hettinger, ND: Healthy Weight, 1997.

Marjolijn K. Bijlefeld and Sharon Zoumbaris
Food and You: A Guide to Healthy Habits for Teens. Westport, CT: Greenwood, 2001.

Lawrence Clayton
Diet Pill Drug Dangers. Springfield, NJ: Enslow, 2001.

Michelle Daum
The Can-Do Eating Plan for Overweight Kids and Teens. New York: Avon, 1997.

Eve Eliot
Insatiable—The Compelling Story of Four Teens, Food, and Its Power. Deerfield Beach, FL: Life Issues, 2001.

Helen Frost and Gail Saunders-Smith	*Fats and Sweets.* Mankato, MN: Capstone, 2000.
Lori Gottlieb	*Stick Figure: A Diary of My Former Self.* New York: Simon and Schuster, 2000.
Cynthia Stamper Graff, Janet Eastman, and Mark C. Smith	*Body Pride: An Action Plan for Teens: Seeking Self-Esteem and Building Better Bodies.* Glendale, CA: Griffin, 1997.
Bill Haduch and Lisa Moore	*Food Rules!* East Rutherford, NJ: Penguin Putnam, 2001.
Marya Hornbacher	*Wasted: A Memoir of Anorexia and Bulimia.* New York: HarperCollins, 1998.
James A. Joseph, Daniel A. Nadeau, and Anne Underwood	*Color Code: A Revolutionary Eating Plan for Optimal Health.* New York: Hyperion, 2002.
Michelle Joy Levine	*I Wish I Were Thin, I Wish I Were Fat: The Reasons We Overeat and What We Can Do About It.* New York: Simon and Schuster, 1999.
Donna Maurer and Jeffrey Sobel	*Interpreting Weight: The Social Management of Fatness and Thinness.* Berlin, Germany: Aldine de Guyter, 1999.
Mimi Nichter	*Fat Talk: What Girls and Their Parents Say About Dieting.* Cambridge, MA: Harvard University Press, 2000.

Carol Emery
Normandi and
Laurelee Roark

Over It. Novato, CA: New World
Library, 2001.

Stephanie Pierson

*Vegetables Rock! A Complete Guide for
Teenage Vegetarians.* New York: Ran-
dom House, 1999.

Jeremy Roberts

Drugs and Dieting. New York: Rosen,
2001.

Sara Shandler

Ophelia Speaks. New York: Harper-
Collins, 1999.

Erica Smith

*Anorexia Nervosa: When Food Is the
Enemy.* New York: Rosen, 1999.

Pamela M. Smith

The Diet Trap. Washington, DC:
Regnery, 2000.

Marilyn Wann

Fat! So? Berkeley, CA: Ten Speed,
1998.

Jonathan Watson

*Male Bodies: Health, Culture, and
Identity.* London: Taylor and Francis,
2000.

Aileen Weintraub

*Everything You Need to Know About
Eating Smart.* New York: Rosen, 2000.

Dorothy F. West

*Nutrition and Fitness: Lifestyle Choices
for Wellness.* Tinley, IL: Goodheart-
Willcox, 1999.

Patsy Westcott

Diet and Nutrition. New York: Raintree
Steck-Vaughn, 2000.

Carrie Latt Wiatt   *Portion Savvy*. New York: Pocket, 1999.

Susan Zannos   *Female Stars of Nutrition and Weight Control*. Bear, DE: Mitchell Lane, 2000.

Periodicals

Janice Arenofsky   "Teens Who Turned Bad Habits into Good Health," *Current Health 2*, May 1997.

Cylin Busby   "Beautiful Girls, Ugly Disease," *Teen*, May 2001.

Dan Cray   "The Low-Carb Diet Craze," *Time*, November 1, 1999.

Cindy Crosscope-   "Male Anorexia Nervosa: A New
Happel et al.   Focus," *Journal of Mental Health Counseling*, October 2000.

Julie K.L. Dam   "Diet Riot," *People Weekly*, June 12, 2000.

Dixie Farley   "On the Teen Scene: Eating Disorders Require Medical Attention," *FDA Consumer*, September 1997.

Nan Kathryn Fuchs   "How to Lose Weight and Keep It Off," *Women's Health Letter*, January 2001.

Michael Fumento   "Busting the Low-Fat Dieting Myth," *Consumers' Research Magazine*, October 1997.

Beth Gooch   "Losing Friends, Losing Weight, Losing
                            Control," *New York Times Upfront*, April
                            30, 2001.

Cynthia Guttman   "Advertising, My Mirror," *UNESCO
                            Courier*, July 2001.

Donald Hensrud   "Fad Diets: All Protein, No Proof," *For-
                            tune*, May 15, 2000.

Thomas Incledon   "Ten Laws of Leanness," *Men's Health*,
                            January 2001.

Beth Israel   "Two Girls Talk About Food, Fat, Bod-
                            ies, and 'Bones,'" *Redbook*, October
                            1997.

Monica Jones   "Scaling Down the Science of Sensible
                            Eating," *American Fitness*, September/
                            October 1997.

Susan McClelland   "Distorted Images: Western Cultures
                            Are Exporting Their Dangerous Obses-
                            sion with Thinness," *Maclean's*, August
                            14, 2000.

Martha Miller and   "Eat Well, Feel Great, Lose Weight,"
Jeanne Ambrose   *Better Homes and Gardens*, June 2000.

Celia Milne   "Pressures to Conform: The Thin
                            Shapely Look Can Be Dangerously Un-
                            realistic," *Maclean's*, January 12, 1998.

Anne Novitt-Morena   "Obesity: What's the Genetic Connec-
                            tion?" *Current Health 2*, February 1998.

| Ellen A. Shur, Mary Sanders, and Hans Steiner | "Dieting and Body Dissatisfaction in Young Children," *Nutrition Research Newsletter*, January 2000. |

Michele Stanten — "Weight Loss Rip-Off or Weight Loss Payoff?" *Prevention*, January 2001.

Beatrice Trum-Hunter — "Eating Disorders: Perilous Compulsions," *Consumers' Research Magazine*, September 1997.

Selene Yeager — "Lose 10, 20, 30 Pounds or More!" *Prevention*, April 1999.

Index

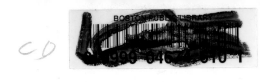